REFLEXOLOGY
AN ILLUSTRATED GUIDE

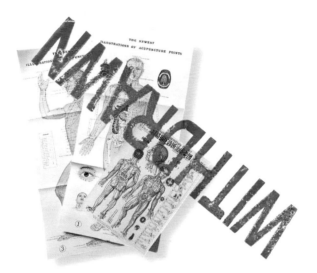

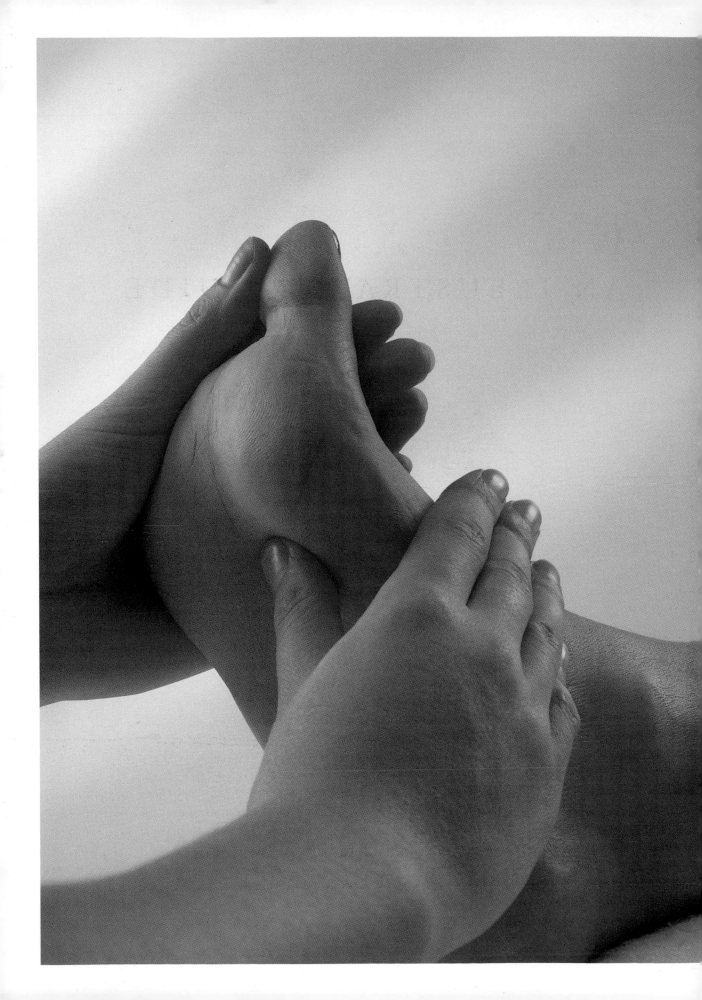

REFLEXOLOGY
AN ILLUSTRATED GUIDE

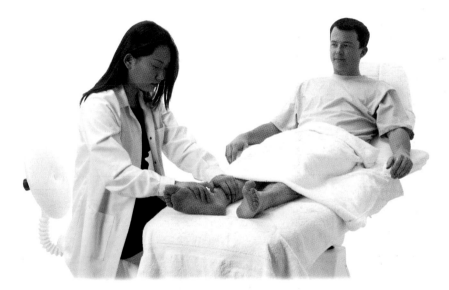

BERYL CRANE

Shaftesbury, Dorset • Boston, Massachusetts • Melbourne, Victoria

© Element Books Limited 1998
Text and techniques © Beryl Crane 1998

First published in Great Britain in 1998 by
ELEMENT BOOKS LIMITED
Shaftesbury, Dorset, SP7 8BP

Published in the USA in 1998 by
ELEMENT BOOKS INC
160 North Washington Street, Boston, MA 02114

Published in Australia in 1998 by
ELEMENT BOOKS
and distributed by Penguin Australia Ltd
487 Maroondah Highway, Ringwood, Victoria 3134

Charts produced by Beryl Crane © 1998

Photographic sessions and techniques supervised
by Beryl Crane

NOTE FROM THE PUBLISHER
*Any information given in this book is not
intended to be taken as a replacement for
medical advice. Any person with a condition
requiring medical attention should consult a
qualified practitioner or therapist.*

Designed and created with
THE BRIDGEWATER BOOK COMPANY LIMITED

ELEMENT BOOKS LIMITED
Senior Commissioning Editor: *Caro Ness*
Managing Editor: *Miranda Spicer*
Production Manager: *Susan Sutterby*

THE BRIDGEWATER BOOK COMPANY
Art Director: KEVIN KNIGHT
Designers: JANE LANAWAY, CHRIS LANAWAY
Managing Editor: ANNE TOWNLEY
Project Editor: CAROLINE EARLE
Picture Research: LYNDA MARSHALL

Printed and bound in Great Britain by Butler and Tanner Ltd.

British Library Cataloguing in Publication
data available

Library of Congress Cataloging-in-Publication
data available

ISBN 1–86204–169–5

Acknowledgments

*The publisher would like to thank
the following for the use of pictures:*
Ancient Art & Architecture Collection: 23R
Bayly School of Reflexology, Whitbourne, Worcs.: 16T
Bridgeman Art Library: 11T, 28T
Dwight Byers, Ingham Publishing, St. Petersburg, Florida: 15T
Hutchison Library: 26T
Image Bank: 10TL, 18C
Images Colour Library: 27C, 78R, 79, 86B
Science Photo Library: 17T, 18B, 82
Werner Forman Archive: 10C

With thanks to:
Clara Bayes, Joseph Harding, Kay Macmullan, Julie Whitaker
for help with photography

Special thanks to:
Carlton Professional, Steyning

Contents

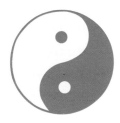

Introduction

THE SENSE OF TOUCH *is very important to us, and we use it instinctively to calm and to alleviate hurt in others, from soothing a crying infant to comforting a friend who has suffered physical or emotional pain. The therapy of reflexology is an extension of these natural gestures. Healing by touch is as old as humanity itself, and pressure or massage (which comes from an Arabic word meaning to "touch" or "palpate") has historically been used as a restorative to health and strength.*

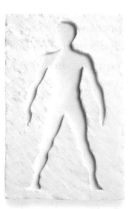

ABOVE *Reflexology stimulates the body's inner healing capabilities.*

There are many different touch or massage therapies, but they are all based on the common principle that for good health, the body's interdependent processes need to be kept in a state of correct balance and flow. When that flow is impeded, a condition of "stagnation" occurs and a particular area then becomes more and more out of balance. Stimulation to the nervous system by touch is believed to restore the natural state of balance.

Reflexology is a type of treatment in which pressure is applied to specific small areas of the skin, mainly the hands and feet. It is a noninvasive, natural therapy that induces a deeply relaxed state, which alleviates tension, mild anxiety, and depression from everyday living. A further effect is that it triggers the body's own inner healing processes. It therefore relieves naturally many medical conditions over a period of time to achieve positive and lasting health benefits. The combination of treatment and relaxation creates a powerful tool and, if used together with skills in counseling and nutritional advice, it provides a total holistic health program.

RIGHT *We use touch instinctively to comfort both physical and emotional pain.*

How to Use this Book

The first sections of this book provide a brief account of the principles and theories of reflexology, and a look at how reflexology has developed over time from its beginnings in the massage and pressure therapies of ancient cultures. We then examine how reflexology exerts its effects by looking at the workings of the nervous system, and how it fits into a contemporary, holistic approach to health and self-maintenance incorporating diet, exercise, and lifestyle.

The sections on the practice of reflexology start by looking at basic pressure techniques, grips, and support holds. A typical treatment session is begun by using preliminary relaxation exercises to relax the limb prior to using pressure treatment, and these are covered next.

The mainstay of reflexology therapy is treatment of the foot and the hand. A complete massage sequence for each is given, covering every body system in turn. In recent years, many reflexologists have also begun to include points on the ear and head, utilizing the meridian theories of Chinese acupuncture and acupressure. These are introduced in separate sections.

An extensive section deals with self-help treatments for common disorders and other problems, and specific points for particular groups such as women, men, children, and the elderly. In each condition, indications are given for reflex points and areas to be used, and additional advice on lifestyle such as dietary tips and useful exercises.

A final section explains what happens when you visit a professional reflexologist, and includes advice on how to find a good therapist, what happens during the treatment, and what effects you can expect during and following the treatment.

BELOW **See how the practice of reflexology may have developed from its origins in the manipulation therapies of the ancient cultures.**

The philosophy behind the modern practice of reflexology is explained in boxed text.

The main text explains the early origins of reflexology, from the time of the Ancient Egyptians.

The text explains precisely how to work the foot or hand for maximum therapeutic benefit.

Step-by-step photography shows you many holds and techniques of reflexology treatment.

Large full-color photographs show the detail of the foot and reflex point being illustrated.

LEFT **Clear and concise step-by-step photography explains the basic techniques of reflexology treatment on the hands, feet, and ears.**

What is Reflexology?

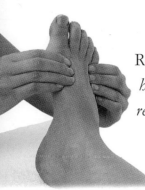

REFLEXOLOGY IS A THERAPY *in which pressure is applied to reflex points on the hands, feet, and also the ears. It is based on the principle that these reflex points are related to the internal organs and glands, and are laid out in the same arrangement as that in the physical body, forming a "map," or microcosm, of it. Pressure or palpation on a reflex point can therefore affect these structures. This treatment helps to stimulate the normal function of the organ involved (for instance, secretion of a hormone or digestive enzyme), and thus aids self-healing, bringing about physical and mental well-being.*

ABOVE *Pressure can be applied to the hands, feet, or ears.*

According to reflexology theory, whose development can be traced back to the beginning of this century, the body is divided longitudinally into 10 zones, five on each side of the midline. These zones run between the toes and the head, and then out to the fingers and thumb (or vice versa). Thus the first zone runs from the great toe (i.e., the big toe) to the center of the head then out to the thumb, the second zone from the second toe to the head, and then to the index finger, and so on. Pressure on reflex points on the foot or hand will affect body organs within the same zone. So, pressing on the thumb or great toe will affect internal structures within this first zone, and will also relieve pain originating anywhere within it, and so on for the other zones.

Reflexology also divides up the foot and hand into four transverse sections. The first transverse zone stretches from the tips to the bases of the toes and fingers, and is related to the neck area and above; it is bounded by a line known as the cervical line. The second transverse zone lies below this, encompassing the ball of the foot and the padded area beneath the fingers, and is related to the organs of the thoracic cavity; it is bounded by a line known as the diaphragm line. The third transverse zone, relating to the abdominal cavity, reaches to, on the foot, a line drawn from the bulge on the outside edge of the foot (anatomically, this is the fifth metatarsal or foot bone notch), and, on the hands, a line from the base of the web between the thumb and index finger; this is called the waistline. The fourth transverse zone is measured from this line down to, on the foot, the bulge found on the side of the ankle, and on the hand, a line running around the wrist at the level of the base of the fleshy part of the thumb; this is the pelvic line.

DIGESTIVE SYSTEM REFLEX POINTS

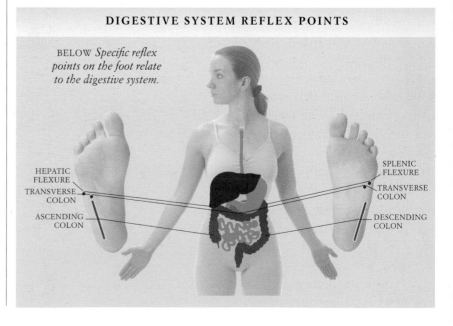

BELOW *Specific reflex points on the foot relate to the digestive system.*

HEPATIC FLEXURE

TRANSVERSE COLON

ASCENDING COLON

SPLENIC FLEXURE

TRANSVERSE COLON

DESCENDING COLON

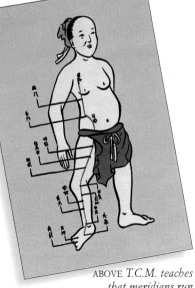

ABOVE *T.C.M. teaches that meridians run through the body.*

Reflexology was developed to work on these zonal energy pathways. In recent years, reflexologists have also begun to incorporate the acupressure techniques of Traditional Chinese Medicine (known as T.C.M.) into their treatment. Although reflexology is based on the theory of zones rather than on the meridian theory of Traditional Chinese Medicine, reflexology treatment does also contact many of the known acupuncture points (*see Appendix Two, p. 136*). Both treatments are based on the principle that specific points can be manipulated to bring about a therapeutic effect in other areas of the body. The meridian theory of T.C.M. is explained later in the book (*see p. 11*).

By applying palpation or alternating pressure on reflex points, a reflexologist first detects areas of imbalance and congestion within the body systems, and then aims to restore the body's natural equilibrium and encourage the body to heal itself at its own pace.

BODY ZONES

According to reflexology theory, the body is divided into ten longitudinal zones that run from the tip of the toes to the head and out to the tips of the fingers, or vice versa. Certain zones are linked to another by energy flow.

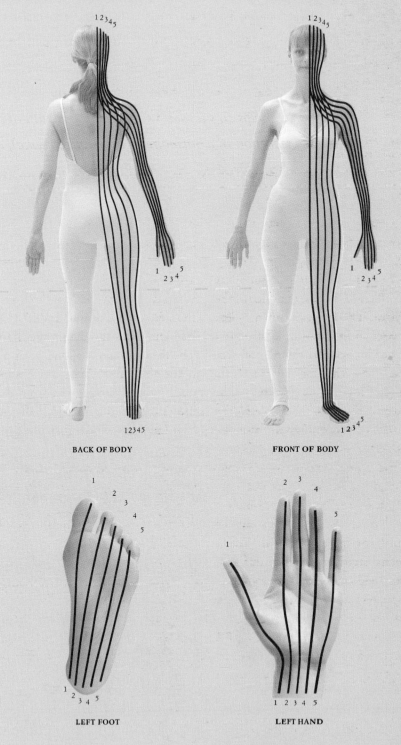

BACK OF BODY

FRONT OF BODY

LEFT FOOT

LEFT HAND

The Origins of Reflexology

THE ROOTS OF REFLEXOLOGY *are found in many different cultures,*
from the tombs of Ancient Egypt to the earliest texts of Traditional Chinese
Medicine. Ancient techniques of pressure to relieve pain were widely used
in earlier times, although the supposition that reflexology as we know
it dates back to ancient times, and that it was one of the secrets of
the Chinese and Egyptians, has never been proven.

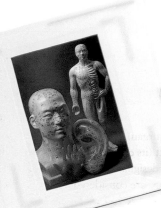

ABOVE *The roots of
modern reflexology can
be traced back to many
different ancient cultures.*

THE MEDITERRANEAN

The art and techniques of massage
and manipulation of the body
largely come from Greece, Rome,
North Africa, and the Arabian
peninsula. They date back many
thousands of years and have been
known from this time to have a
profound and positive effect on the
health of the recipient. Known
as the "father of medicine,"
Hippocrates (*c.* 460–377 B.C.E.),
a physician of
Ancient Greece,
spoke of rubbing
and manipulation
in order to relieve
pain in the joints.

RIGHT *Hippocrates, the
famous Greek physician,
advocated the use of
touch to relieve swollen
and painful joints.*

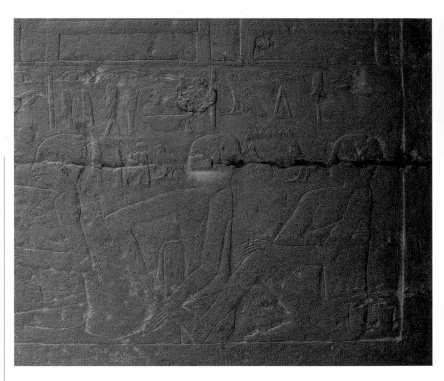

ABOVE *The Ancient Egyptians used
massage and manipulation to relieve
painful conditions.*

EGYPT

The ancient Egyptians also used
massage daily. It is in one of their
tombs that the first depictions of
some sort of treatment of the toes
and fingers have been found. In
Saqqara, the tomb of "Ankhm'ahor,"
known as the "physician's tomb,"
and dating back to the Sixth Dynasty
(2423–2263 B.C.E.), is believed by
some to illustrate a reflexology
treatment. One relief shows massage
or manipulation to the foot or leg
and shoulder, which could indicate a
form of pressure therapy or
reflexology treatment being applied
on the hands and feet, with
accompanying massage to the
legs and back.

CHINA

The traditional system of medicine practiced by the Chinese people, which is generally known as Traditional Chinese Medicine (or T.C.M.), is founded upon empirical observations. It is the result of practical experiences dating back for thousands of years. It has many branches, including herbal medicine, moxa (burning sticks made of rolled herbs, used to heat specific body areas), acupuncture needling, acupressure, thumb and finger pressure, and massage, and qigong (pronounced "chi kung" – a healing exercise combining slow movements, breathing, and mental focusing). Underlying all of these techniques is a common theory with distinct features.

This theory is a principle termed "Qi" or "Chi," which has various meanings, including "vital force," "inner vital energy," "air," and "breath." Qi is essential to life, and a deficiency or an imbalance (caused by a blockage in one part of the body) is the root cause of ill-health. All T.C.M. methods aim to unblock any "stasis" (stagnation) of Qi, in order to reinstate its natural flow.

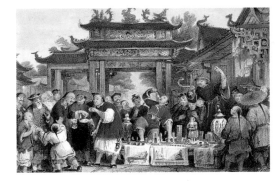

LEFT *Traditional Chinese Medicine (T.C.M.) is an ancient form of healing that dates back thousands of years.*

YIN AND YANG

Another idea underlying T.C.M. philosophy is that of Yin and Yang, two universal principles of polarity. Yin is the principle embodied by femininity, darkness, night, coldness, softness, receptivity, descent, interior, while Yang is the opposite principle of masculinity, light, day, heat, hardness, activity, ascent, exterior. These two principles, while opposites, also complement each other and are mutually dependent. The correct balance between these two opposites, the negative and the positive, is necessary to maintain good health; the same principle of balance is applied in reflexology treatment.

Within the body, the hollow organs and their associated circulatory or distribution systems – for instance,

YIN/YANG SYMBOL

the stomach (organ) with the intestinal tract (its distribution system) – are designated Yang, and the solid organs are considered Yin. The Yang organs are considered to transform and transport substances that have been taken into the body, while the Yin organs store substances. The Yang organs are the Stomach, Small Intestine, Large Intestine, Bladder, Gallbladder, and Triple Burner; the Yin organs are the Heart, Liver, Spleen/Pancreas, Lungs, Kidney, and Pericardium. (Note that the Chinese "organs" do not correspond exactly to the anatomical organs – for instance, the Chinese "Kidney" includes the adrenal glands – so by convention they are capitalized to avoid confusion.)

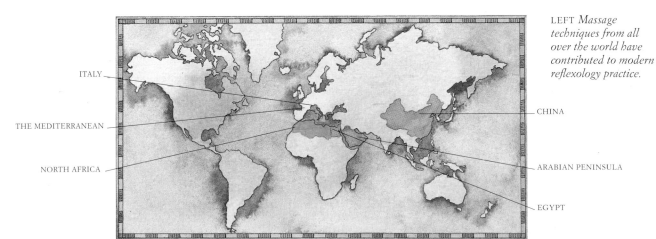

LEFT *Massage techniques from all over the world have contributed to modern reflexology practice.*

ITALY

THE MEDITERRANEAN

NORTH AFRICA

CHINA

ARABIAN PENINSULA

EGYPT

THE MERIDIANS

These ideas gave rise to the meridian theory. The Chinese often used the ideas of clear and stagnant water as an analogy for the circulation of Qi in the body, and meridians were considered to be channels of Qi that were like rivers of water running through the body. This idea was elaborated to include the concept that there were also "reservoirs" of Qi that could be utilized in times of stress (so people with ample reserves of Qi had greater stamina), and that when Qi was prevented from flowing properly, and carrying away toxins (known as "pathogenic factors" in T.C.M.) to the organs of elimination, then it produced an effect similar to the accumulation of debris and stagnation of water, with ill-health the inevitable result. In addition, there were certain points along these meridians where it was particularly easy to adjust and balance the flow of Qi, called "acupuncture points" (or acupoints); these points functioned somewhat like the lock-gates in a canal, allowing practitioners to increase or decrease the amount and quality of the Qi in a particular meridian as necessary.

Each of the organs mentioned previously (*see p. 11*) had an associated meridian. These 12 "organ meridians" were designated Yin or Yang depending on the organ with which they originated from and were connected. Six of these (three Yin and three Yang) connect the fingers and the upper body; the three Yin meridians (Lung, Heart, Pericardium) descend from the chest to the fingers, while the three Yang meridians (Large Intestine, Small Intestine, Triple Burner) ascend from the fingers to the face.

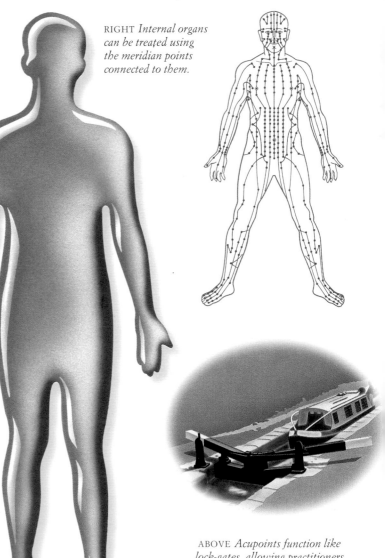

RIGHT *Internal organs can be treated using the meridian points connected to them.*

RIGHT *In T.C.M., Qi is said to flow through the body's meridians like rivers of water.*

ABOVE *Reservoirs of Qi can be used in times of stress. People with good reserves are said to have greater stamina.*

ABOVE *Acupoints function like lock-gates, allowing practitioners to increase or decrease the amount of Qi as necessary.*

A further six (again three Yin and three Yang) connect the toes and the upper body; the Yin meridians (the Liver, Spleen, and Kidney) ascend from the toes to the chest area, while the Yang meridians (the Stomach, Bladder, and Gallbladder) descend from the face to the toes. In addition, there were other channels that performed a more general regulatory function, or were considered "reservoirs" of Qi; these were termed "vessels." Two of the most important vessels are the Governor Vessel (Yang), which runs up the spine and over the head to the upper gum, and regulates and harmonizes the Yang meridians, and the Conception Vessel (Yin), which runs up the front of the body to the lower jaw, and regulates and harmonizes the Yin meridians. Detailed meridian maps can be found at the back of the book (*see Appendix Two, p. 136*).

Each of the internal organs can be treated medically by using the points on the meridian connected with it. Treating the points at the beginning and end of the meridians were believed to be relatively powerful in effect. It can immediately be seen that treating the feet, hands, and head would be considered particularly beneficial, so this is in complete agreement with reflexology theory.

In addition to treatment of these areas, auricular (ear) therapy also has a long history in China. Ear acupuncture has been used there for thousands of years. Auricular diagnostic and therapeutic methods were first used and documented about around 200 B.C.E, and at one time there were over 230 different acupoints in the ear being used.

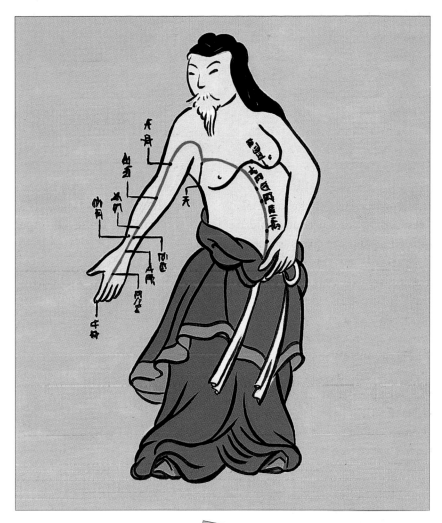

ABOVE AND RIGHT *In T.C.M., each organ of the body has a meridian line that acts on Yin or Yang energy.*

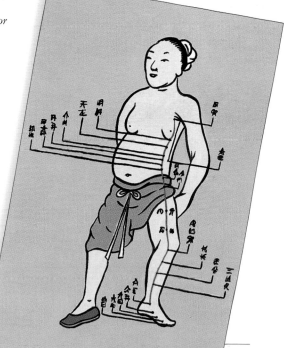

Early Reflexologists

ALTHOUGH THE PARALLELS *with early pressure therapies are fascinating, reflexology itself developed entirely separately. The precise techniques of modern reflexology can be traced back to research on nervous reflex actions over 100 years ago. It was based on discoveries made in Europe and the United States during the late 1800s relating to the mechanics of reflex action within the nervous system.*

The 19th century was a fertile period of discovery. Physicians and scientists at that time began to study abnormal foot reflexes that were not evident in healthy individuals. These were found to indicate damage to, or absence of, a particular nerve or nerve tract. They were thus a means of furthering scientific knowledge of the nervous system, as these reflex actions indicated the pathways of nerve action taking place in the body. From these findings, the basic principle of reflexology was developed. This principle is that pressure to particular skin areas stimulates certain nerve reflexes, thus sending a message to particular areas of the brain concerned with particular functions (*see pp. 18–22*).

WILLIAM FITZGERALD (1872–1942)

Reflexology, as it is now known, originated with the zone therapy of Dr. William Fitzgerald M.D. of Hartford, Connecticut, an eminent U.S. physician who graduated from the University of Vermont in 1895 and worked first at the Boston City Hospital, then at the Central London Ear, Nose, and Throat (E.N.T.) Hospital in England (1902). This was followed by a further period in an E.N.T. hospital in Vienna alongside Professor Politzer and Professor Otto Chiari, who were well known in the medical world at the beginning of the 20th century. He then became the senior nose and throat surgeon at St. Francis Hospital, Hartford, Connecticut for several years. It was here that he made his findings of "zone therapy," as it was then called, known to the medical field.

Dr. Fitzgerald never explained in his writings how he arrived at the concept of "zone therapy." However, one theory is that, while working, he discovered that pressing firmly over certain points on the toes and hands and other parts of the body caused a type of

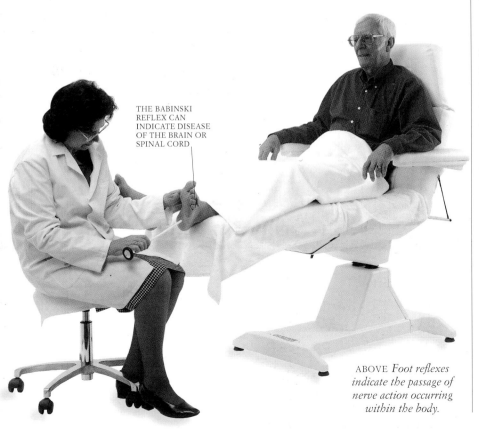

THE BABINSKI REFLEX CAN INDICATE DISEASE OF THE BRAIN OR SPINAL CORD

ABOVE *Foot reflexes indicate the passage of nerve action occurring within the body.*

localized anesthesia. This was sufficient to enable him to perform minor operations on the nose and throat without using cocaine and other local analgesics. By experimenting, he found that applying pressure, either over the bony eminences (e.g., joints) or within zones corresponding longitudinally with the site of the injury, he could not only relieve pain, but, if the pressure were firm enough, induce an anesthetic effect, often somehow removing the cause of the pain.

Dr. Fitzgerald published his first book in 1917 with the help of Dr. Edwin Bowers, a colleague who christened the technique "zone therapy." The title of his book was *Zone Therapy, or Relieving Pain at Home*. In it, he related all his important findings and theories, and in particular the division of the body into 10 longitudinal zones (*see p. 8*). He also showed a link between each of the internal organs and particular zones. He advocated pressure applied to particular fingers or toes to alleviate pain in specific sites or zones. Following the publication of Dr. Fitzgerald's findings, interest in his theories became widespread and the squeezing of fingers or toes was popularly used to alleviate many minor complaints and disorders.

RIGHT *The works of the pioneer reflexologists are still very much used by modern practitioners.*

JOSEPH SHELBY-RILEY
EARLY 1900s

Dr. Fitzgerald taught many colleagues, who in turn also wrote books developing the theory of reflexology. One of these was Dr. Joe Shelby-Riley, a chiropractor who published several books. These include *Zone Therapy Simplified* (1919) and *Science and Practice of Chiropractic with Allied Sciences* (1925), in which he included material on zone therapy.

In Dr. Shelby-Riley's books, he not only worked with the zones and their reflexes, but also included a few auricular and facial points. He recommended ear points for cold feet, paralysis, goiter, thyroid problems, and also for earache or deafness. For constipation, he recommended firm pressure on the chin and other facial points.

ABOVE *Dr. Shelby-Riley, one of the key figures in early reflexology.*

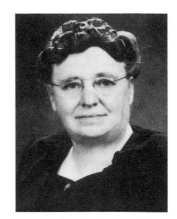

ABOVE *Eunice Ingham, the U.S. author of two classic reflexology books.*

EUNICE INGHAM
(1889–1974)

During the 1930s, the theory of reflexology was further refined into its modern form by Eunice Ingham in the United States.

In 1938, she published *Stories the Feet Can Tell*. This was followed in 1945 with a revised book entitled *Stories the Feet Have Told*. These classic texts form the basis of modern reflexology, and are still very much in use by practitioners.

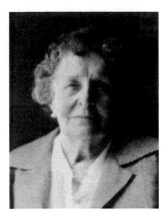

ABOVE *Doreen Bayly took the practice of reflexology to the U.K.*

DOREEN BAYLY
(1900–1979)

Reflexology was taken to the U.K. in 1966 by Doreen Bayly when she returned from the U.S. after training with Eunice Ingham. In 1978, she wrote *Reflexology Today*. Many of her former students have become practitioners or principals of their own schools.

PAUL NOGIER 1950s

In addition to pressure applied to the feet and hands, more recently the ears have become another way of applying stimulation to the body. This is partly because the techniques of ear acupuncture have been brought to the West. In addition, there was a second separate development in auricular therapy, which stemmed from a French practitioner, Dr. Paul Nogier. In the early 1950s, he introduced a theory that proposed the concept of an "inverted fetus" shape lying within the ear, a theory that he published in 1972. According to this theory, within the ear is a representation of the human body, similar in shape to the inverted fetus (i.e., in an upside-down position), with the head laying near the lower lobe, the feet and hands toward the upper rim, and the body in between. There is a corresponding pattern of auricular points, each of which, like the reflex points of the foot and hand, relate to the internal organs and can be used by practitioners to treat related complaints.

THE FETUS' BODY LIES BETWEEN THE UPPER RIM AND LOWER LOBE

HEAD CORRESPONDS TO LOWER EAR LOBE

HANDS AND FEET CORRESPOND TO UPPER RIM OF EAR

RIGHT *The points on the ear are said to correspond to those of an inverted fetus.*

C.2,500 B.C.E.	C.2,300 B.C.E.	C.460–377	1582	1886	1892
Acupuncture is developed by the Chinese. Needles are inserted at specific points along the meridians throughout the body to bring about harmony and a balance of "life forces" or Qi.	The tomb of Ankhm'ahor in Saqqara in Egypt is known as the physician's tomb due to the marvelous portrayal of medicine on its walls, including foot and hand treatments.	Hippocrates, the Greek physician, was one of the first to advocate massaging or rubbing an area of the body as a form of therapeutic relaxation.	Two eminent physicians from Leipzig, Dr. Adamus and Dr. A'tatis, publish a book on zone therapy.	Vladimir Mikhailovich Bekhterev *(1857–1927)* uses experimental methods of reflexology on animals and later humans in Russia.	In France, Dr. Joseph François Felix Babinski ascertained the plantar reflex. By using a blunt, pointed object on the lateral side of the sole of the foot, a reflex is obtained. A certain response could indicate disease of the brain or spinal cord.

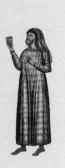

REFLEXOLOGY TODAY

Reflexology as it is now practiced has developed into a precise technique of palpation and pressure that is far removed from its early simplistic beginnings. Since the 1980s, complementary medicine, and reflexology specifically (over 100 books have now been written on the subject), has become a growth area. Research by neuroscientists on related disciplines, such as acupuncture, has revealed how nervous fibers and brain pathways are stimulated by physical methods, and research on the clinical effectiveness has also been initiated.

Practitioners have developed precise techniques and locations for applying pressure; some practitioners take into account

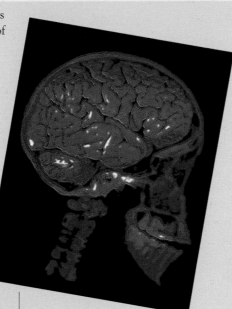

ABOVE *Modern research as shown how physical manipulation can stimulate nerve pathways in the brain.*

the meridian theories of T.C.M. in order to provide an integrated and holistic therapy.

At the same time, auricular therapy using a combination of Dr. Nogier's theory and T.C.M. has become extremely well known. Particular useages, for example smoking addiction, have become increasingly popular with the public.

Reflexology at all levels requires an extensive knowledge of the body systems, and many reflexology organizations have formed registers of qualified practitioners. Reflexologists in the UK have worked towards achieving government recognition. A National Training Organisation has now been formed, and funding will help insure that high standards of training are maintained.

1893	1904	1917	1938	1955	1966
he English eurologist Sir enry Head 861–1940) ublished research onfirming the direct lationship between essure applied to e skin and its effect n the internal gans.	The Russian Ivan Petrovitch Pavlov *(1849–1936)* receives the Nobel Prize for showing that there is a direct association between a stimulus and a response to a reflex action.	Dr. William Fitzgerald *(1872–1942)* published his findings on zone therapy in the U.S. He outlined a totally holistic method of healing by pressure to specific areas of the hand, foot, and other areas of the body. Dr. Joe Shelby-Riley, an American naturopath, publishes a number of books on zone therapy.	In the U.S., Eunice Ingham *(1889–1974)*, a pupil of Joe Riley, publishes her first book, *Stories The Feet Can Tell.*	Harry Bond Bressler publishes a book on zone therapy in the U.S. In it, he pays credit to William Fitzgerald and Edwin F. Bowers, who collaborated with Fitzgerald on his first book.	Doreen Bayly, who trained with Eunice Ingham, returns to the United Kingdom to instruct many of today's early European practitioners of reflexology.

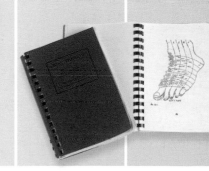

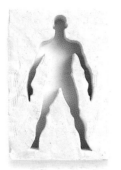

How Reflexology Works

MANY BOOKS HAVE ATTEMPTED *some explanation of the precise workings of reflexology, and although much more is now understood about the nerve pathways involved, much still remains to be elucidated. The basic premise of reflexology is that the stimulation applied somehow acts to clear nervous and tissue congestion, removing accumulated toxins from them and encouraging the body's own innate healing ability.*

ABOVE *Reflexology aims to clear the body of accumulated toxins.*

ENERGY

Every living thing needs energy. Most natural energy on our planet comes from the sun, and this energy is transferred to growing plants and from them to animals and humans. The energy that our bodies require is therefore obtained from our food. It is needed in order to carry out essential processes such as movement, reproduction, and growth; even sleeping and resting require energy, as we still use oxygen and produce carbon dioxide during these periods of relative inactivity.

Our bodies use different forms of energy for different functions. The nervous system uses both electrical energy and chemical energy to send its signals from the sensory receptors at the body surface along the nerve fibers to the spinal cord or brain, and back down other nerve fibers to the muscles or end organs such as digestive and endocrine glands (*see pp. 20–21*). Information travels by electrical means along a nerve cell, and chemically between the cells. This energy follows set paths, and this statement remains true whether we think in terms of the transmission of a nerve impulse

ABOVE *The natural energy on our planet comes primarily from the sun.*

along the nerve fibers or whether we believe in the T.C.M. idea of transmission of Qi down the meridian pathways (*see pp. 12–13*). Whichever system reflexology treatment is actually utilizing, it is fundamentally a method of accessing and altering information in the body's energy transmission system via the many reflex points on the feet or hands.

RIGHT *One of the functions of the cells in the cerebral cortex is to interpret sensory impulses.*

WHAT IS A REFLEX?

Any physical therapy involves stimulation to the touch-sensitive sensory cells on the surface of the skin, called receptor cells. Stimulation of the reflex points on the skin sends messages from these cells through nerve pathways to the control centers inside the body, which send other messages back to the muscles or internal organs. In a reflex pathway, the message follows a relatively simple circuit, in which the spinal and lower, primitive brain centers receive the message and send out a directive for the response required straight back to the muscles or internal organ. The higher, conscious control centers in the brain are not always involved.

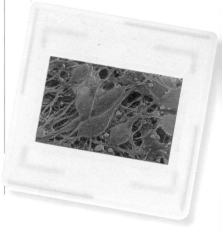

Thus we are frequently not consciously aware of the response we have made. The advantage of this type of response is that it is much faster than sending a message through to the conscious part of the brain, as this could take several seconds to decide on a response, which may be fatal in an emergency. Thus a painful stimuli such as a burn will bring about a reflex of withdrawing the body part involved; it is a rapid, automatic, involuntary activity that can have a great survival value in a serious emergency.

The medical profession often uses these reflexes to help in diagnosis. Physicians test for a reflex called the "plantar reflex" by drawing a blunt-pointed instrument along the outside (lateral) edge of the sole of the foot, from heel to toe.

The normal response would be a downward bunching movement of the toes. An upward movement of the big toes is often a sensitive indication of disease in the brain or spinal cord. This reflex is also known as the Babinski reflex.

Unconscious reflex actions are extremely important and are used continually by the body in everyday actions that do not require conscious decisions. For example, they regulate the activity of the internal organs, such as those of the digestive system, and continually adjust the tone of muscles, including those used in posture. It is probably for this reason that reflexology has such a dynamic effect on all the spinal nerves of the vertebrae improving all back and neck-related problems, and also digestion.

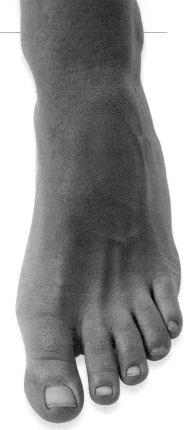

ABOVE *Reflexes on the sole and outside edge of the foot determine brain or spinal cord malfunction.*

REFLEX ACTIONS

RIGHT *Our reflex actions are vital in emergency situations, for example if we burn ourselves.*

PRIMITIVE BRAIN CENTERS RECEIVE MESSAGE

HAND FEELS PAIN

BRAIN SENDS DIRECTIVE FOR RESPONSE STRAIGHT BACK TO MUSCLES

HAND IS QUICKLY REMOVED FROM DANGER

THE NERVOUS SYSTEM

The nervous system is generally divided into a number of parts. First, there is the division into the central nervous system (the brain and the spinal cord) and the peripheral nervous system, which includes the 43 pairs of nerves that arise from them. Sensory nerves transmit impulses from the periphery of the body to the spinal cord, these impulses may or may not pass to the brain or to a connecter neurone of a reflex arc. The motor nerve fibers transmit impulses from the brain through the spinal cord to organs such as skeletal muscles, the smooth muscle and glands of the involuntary nervous system. This is the autonomic nervous system (supplying the glands, heart muscle, and muscle of the internal organs). Reflexology treatment exerts one of its effects mainly through the autonomic nervous system, balancing the opposing actions of its two main subdivisions – the sympathetic branch, whose impulses tend to dominate when the body is in a demanding, stressful situation (for instance, increasing the heart rate and stimulating epinephrine (adrenaline) production, and the parasympathetic branch, whose impulses tend to dominate when the body is calm and peaceful, and promote digestive activity (for instance, reducing the heart rate and stimulating production of digestive juices). Since it is the sympathetic branch that is frequently overactive in our stressful modern lives, it is most often the action of the parasympathetic nervous system that is increased by the treatment. Therefore, when giving reflexology treatment, a person's heart rate often decreases.

The autonomic nervous system was given its name because it was originally thought to be self-regulating and independent from the other parts of the nervous system. Later this was found to be not entirely true. Although most of its responses are involuntary, some meditation and exercise systems appear to develop some degree of conscious influence over it (for instance, yoga, meditation, and the Chinese exercises of Tai Chi and qigong). Biofeedback techniques, which use electrical monitoring equipment to detect and relay physiological changes, have the same effect, and have been used, for instance, to train migraine sufferers to alter the blood flow in their heads.

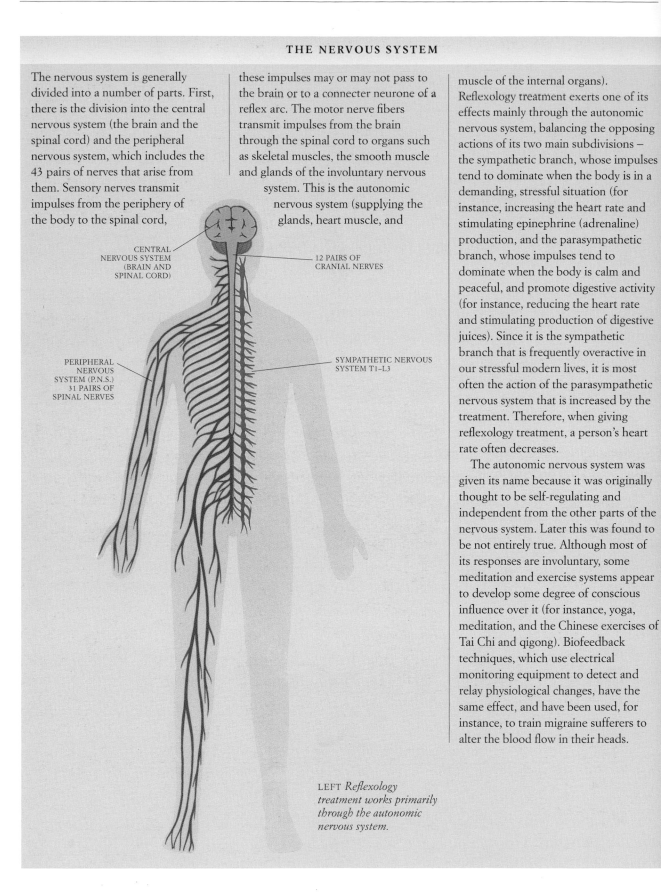

CENTRAL
NERVOUS SYSTEM
(BRAIN AND
SPINAL CORD)

12 PAIRS OF
CRANIAL NERVES

PERIPHERAL
NERVOUS
SYSTEM (P.N.S.)
31 PAIRS OF
SPINAL NERVES

SYMPATHETIC NERVOUS
SYSTEM T1–L3

LEFT *Reflexology treatment works primarily through the autonomic nervous system.*

FUNCTIONS OF THE AUTONOMIC NERVOUS SYSTEM

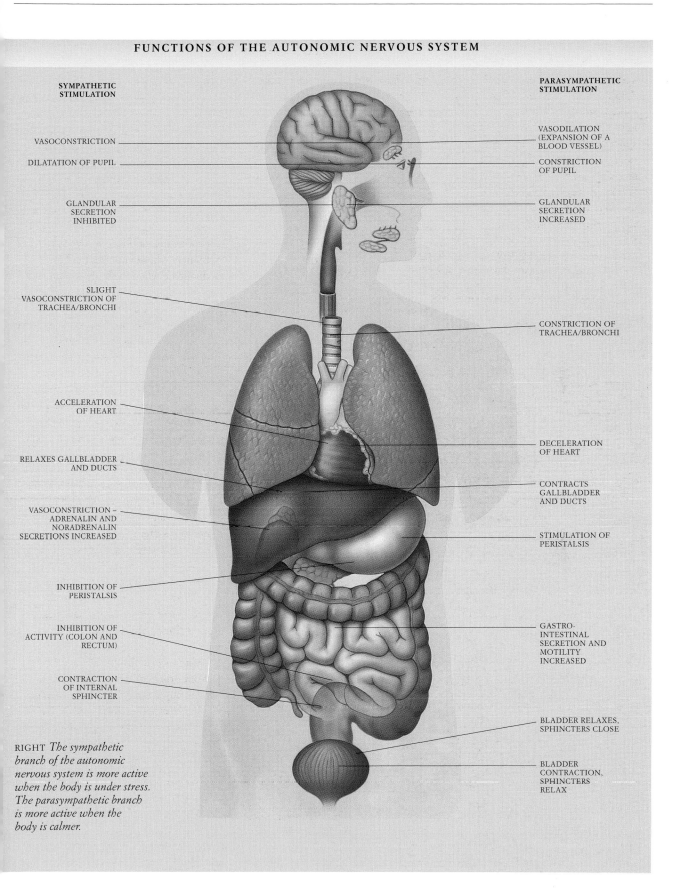

SYMPATHETIC STIMULATION

VASOCONSTRICTION

DILATATION OF PUPIL

GLANDULAR SECRETION INHIBITED

SLIGHT VASOCONSTRICTION OF TRACHEA/BRONCHI

ACCELERATION OF HEART

RELAXES GALLBLADDER AND DUCTS

VASOCONSTRICTION – ADRENALIN AND NORADRENALIN SECRETIONS INCREASED

INHIBITION OF PERISTALSIS

INHIBITION OF ACTIVITY (COLON AND RECTUM)

CONTRACTION OF INTERNAL SPHINCTER

PARASYMPATHETIC STIMULATION

VASODILATION (EXPANSION OF A BLOOD VESSEL)

CONSTRICTION OF PUPIL

GLANDULAR SECRETION INCREASED

CONSTRICTION OF TRACHEA/BRONCHI

DECELERATION OF HEART

CONTRACTS GALLBLADDER AND DUCTS

STIMULATION OF PERISTALSIS

GASTRO-INTESTINAL SECRETION AND MOTILITY INCREASED

BLADDER RELAXES, SPHINCTERS CLOSE

BLADDER CONTRACTION, SPHINCTERS RELAX

RIGHT *The sympathetic branch of the autonomic nervous system is more active when the body is under stress. The parasympathetic branch is more active when the body is calmer.*

21

HORMONES AND NEUROTRANSMITTERS

The overall commander of the autonomic nervous system is a part of the brain that is called the hypothalamus, a small area of the forebrain that also regulates the sensations of thirst, hunger, and temperature, and so moderates our levels of food and water intake. It is also involved in regulating sleep patterns and is connected to our emotional activity.

This brain center also governs a gland in the brain called the pituitary, which is a "master gland" that secretes many hormones (chemicals that are released into the blood and balance the levels of important blood compounds, such as sugars and salts, and regulate processes such as growth, reproduction, and responses to stress). It also produces "releasing hormones," which control the activities of other glands, such as the thyroid gland in the throat, and therefore the release of yet other hormones. Imbalance in these hormones can lead directly to a decline in our state of health – refer to the Endocrine System (*see pp. 50–51*). So, if reflexology can rebalance the activity of the hypothalamus through its action on the autonomic nervous system, it is acting at a very deep level to remove an underlying cause of a problem.

An essential part of the working of the nervous system is a group of chemicals that are known as neurotransmitters. The task of these chemicals is to carry over transmission of nerve signals from one nerve cell (neurone) to the next. They may be either excitory (stimulating action) or inhibitory (preventing action). In the nerve endings of the sympathetic nervous system, a neurotransmitter called norepinephrine (noradrenaline) is released; this constricts blood vessels, and therefore tends to increase the blood pressure, and in cardiac muscle quickens and strengthens the heartbeat. In the parasympathetic nervous system, a

HORMONE PRODUCERS

Hormones are the chemical messengers present in our body that control the rate at which glands and other organs work. The pituitary, or master gland, is located in the brain. It controls many of the main endocrine glands. The hypothalamus is also found in the brain.

BRAIN

BELOW *Both the pituitary gland and hypothalamus are centrally located, close to the brain stem.*

PITUITARY GLAND

HYPOTHALAMUS

BRAIN STEM

CEREBELLUM

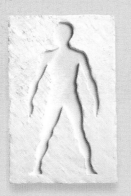

ABOVE *Hormones control many of the body's activities, including metabolism, growth, and sexual reproduction.*

NEUROTRANSMITTERS

Nerve cells (neurons) respond to stimuli by transmitting an electrical impulse. This signal travels down the axon and releases a chemical (known as a neurotransmitter) from the terminals at the axon's end. This in turn may transmit the signal to another neuron.

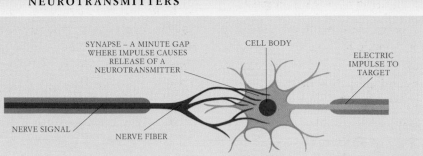

SYNAPSE – A MINUTE GAP WHERE IMPULSE CAUSES RELEASE OF A NEUROTRANSMITTER

CELL BODY

ELECTRIC IMPULSE TO TARGET

NERVE SIGNAL

NERVE FIBER

chemical called acetylcholine is released, which has the opposite effect. A neurotransmitter called serotonin, in the central nervous system, is related to our sleep cycles. There are now known to be over 50 different neurotransmitter substances. One that is important in pain regulation is called substance P; it is found in the brain and spinal cord and is thought to stimulate the perception of pain. So methods such as reflexology and acupuncture, which are effective in stopping pain, may be blocking its release. Or they may be triggering the release of other substances, known as endorphins, which are natural opiate-like substances that inhibit transmission of pain impulses.

MERIDIANS AND NERVES

Many of the Chinese meridians follow the pathways of major nerves. Refer to Appendix Two for detailed meridian maps (*see pp.136–140*). These pathways connect a number of structures along their course, including bones lying very close to the peripheral nerves and muscles attaching to these bones, as well as organs, arteries, and veins. Therefore, we can see that acupuncture, by activating nerve fibers, can potentially affect all of these other structures. Dr. Fitzgerald's original discovery about pain inhibition resulted from his applying pressure over a bone; since the nerves lie very close to the bones, we can also see that reflexology may be working by this very same mechanism.

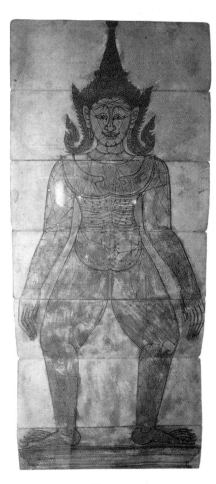

ABOVE *Illustration from a 16th-century Tibetan manuscript on the art of massage. Many of the meridians reflect the pathways of the major nerves in the body.*

LEFT *Reflexology may stimulate the release of endorphins, which inhibit pain impulses.*

The Holistic Approach

THE TERM "HOLISTIC" *is taken from the Greek word "holas," meaning "whole."*
Holism incorporates mind, body, and spirit. Any health problem, whether the
symptoms are primarily physical or mental, is in fact a condition of the whole person.
Social factors also have to be taken into account in any illness, as emotional stress and
mental strain all contribute to ill-health. Similarly, physical injury and illness
precipitate mental symptoms such as depression. Holistic medicine demands that we be
open to a whole spectrum of therapies and practices of health maintenance. Everyone
should therefore include with their reflexology treatment some principles of self-care,
self-healing, and practices for the prevention of ill-health.

It is in everyone's interest to become more aware of both the workings of their internal systems and their feelings. It is well worthwhile also to develop an understanding and awareness of the body's self-healing ability. The body naturally heals itself every day. For instance, when you cut yourself, the body's innate power draws and knits together tissue and heals the wound. The body generally has a great capacity for recovery, provided that its systems are not overloaded or otherwise abused in some way. The tradition of natural healing is to use only the simplest, most natural means to support the body in its self-renewal. It uses adjustments to lifestyle such as diet and exercise to boost

RIGHT *Holistic therapies treat the whole person – mind, body, and spirit – to insure total well-being.*

the vitality and encourage the removal of toxins and impurities that clog up the system and prevent optimal working. Reflexology treatment encourages a generally healthier and fitter body by facilitating the proper functioning of the nervous and circulatory systems, enabling the supply of nutrients and oxygen to reach the whole body. So it is, therefore, a physical therapy that fits well within this natural tradition and philosophy.

According to the natural healing tradition, disease manifests because the body has been ill-treated in some way; it is often our daily repetitive habits that are our own undoing. Yet how many people are aware of the extent to which, by making simple everyday adjustments to their habits, they can help their general health? There are three fundamental golden rules of natural healing that should be included in any health program; these include adopting a nutritious diet, maintaining good habits of posture and taking regular exercise, and developing a well-balanced mental outlook.

RULE 1

The first rule of healthy living is to feed the insides of the body properly. Nutrition is a basic step to improving your inner environment, and a good diet helps to stave off disease. In addition, understanding how your digestive system operates helps you to adopt practices that improve your digestion.

A good diet means a balanced diet, containing all the natural nutrients in the right quantities to provide for the daily functioning of the body without either depleting or increasing the body's stores of nutrients. It includes both the macronutrients such as proteins, fats, carbohydrates (for example, sugars, starch), some minerals, such as calcium, and water, and the micronutrients, such as vitamins and trace minerals (e.g., chromium). However, an incorrect diet, like, for example, eating lots of processed and refined foods, such as excess sugar (which is a dead carbohydrate and has no nutritional benefits whatsoever), can deplete the body's stores of essential nutrients and leave you lacking in vitality.

Eating healthily includes avoiding overeating; eat only sufficient food to keep you healthy and provide enough energy for everyday needs. Many foods require a lot of body energy to digest, so overeating, as well as eating the wrong foods, can slow your body systems down, leaving you feeling tired and lethargic. Refer to Basic Nutrition (*see pp. 28–31*).

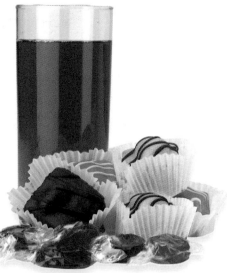

ABOVE *Avoid too much refined food, such as sugar, in your diet, as it has little nutritional value.*

BELOW *A balanced diet is one of the key elements to maintaining a healthy body.*

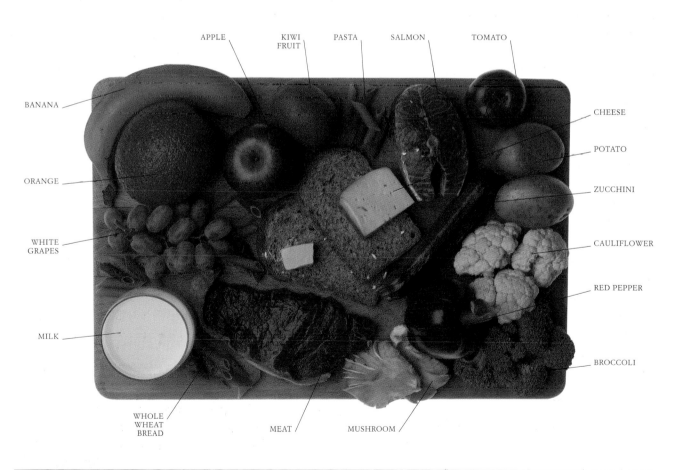

APPLE — KIWI FRUIT — PASTA — SALMON — TOMATO — BANANA — CHEESE — ORANGE — POTATO — ZUCCHINI — WHITE GRAPES — CAULIFLOWER — RED PEPPER — MILK — BROCCOLI — WHOLE WHEAT BREAD — MEAT — MUSHROOM

RULE 2

Become aware of the importance to your health of correct posture, breathing, and exercise. If you are tense, this inhibits your breathing as your diaphragm does not expand and contract properly, your circulation is then impeded, and this robs the tissues of vital oxygen. Relaxation and meditation, as well as many physical activities (climbing stairs, walking, jogging, and many sports) encourage you to breath more deeply.

Take regular exercise daily; brisk walking just for 20 minutes per day is enough to make your heart muscle stronger and improve stamina. Moderate exercise keeps the joints, ligaments, tendons, and muscles strong. It can also help your mood and improve your self-confidence. Be aware, though, that different types and intensities of exercise have different effects. For instance, to improve muscle strength you need to do a program of weight training, but this is anaerobic exercise and does not necessarily protect your heart. For this, you need to do sustained, aerobic exercise. Exercising too hard can have a negative effect on your immune system. Gentle or moderate exercise that does not

ABOVE *Regular Tai Chi exercises will help maintain flexibility and balance.*

wear you out is now thought to be a better option. Slow, rhythmic exercise such as walking, or Tai Chi, can maintain joint flexibility and balance, and prevent osteoporosis as you age. Remember, however, to keep it up – the moment you do not use it you lose it, because the improved physiological functioning quickly reverts back to its original level.

STAND TALL

DON'T ARCH YOUR BACK

RELAX

CHECK YOUR POSTURE

Posture can be checked very easily. Stand with your back against a wall and try to stand tall – there should be no room to put your hand between the small of your back and the wall.

LEFT *Correct posture will help you to breathe more efficiently. Insure that you do not arch your back and stiffen.*

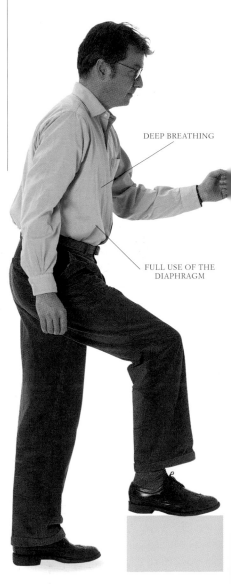

DEEP BREATHING

FULL USE OF THE DIAPHRAGM

RIGHT *Physical activity, such as climbing the stairs, encourages full use of the diaphragm.*

RULE 3

Become aware of what is going on in your mind. You should try to cultivate a positive outlook, as negative thought processes and emotional reactions can affect our nerve force, thereby creating nervous disorders. Changing negative thought habits is the basis of a psychological therapy known as "cognitive therapy." Improper care of the body includes nervous exhaustion, overwork, worry and excess anxiety, and inadequate sleep and relaxation. You should have a break from a constant work routine and find time to relax both mentally and physically, and this includes giving yourself a change of surroundings. Otherwise, many disorders may manifest themselves, including digestive disorders, asthma, panic attacks, anxiety, and depression. Conversely, when a therapy such as reflexology is applied to the physical body, the process of cleansing that takes place allows not only long-standing accumulated body toxins to be released, but also long-standing and deep emotions of anger and grief to surface. This is all part of the cleansing work.

BELOW *Take time to relax mentally and physically, preferably in pleasant, tranquil surroundings.*

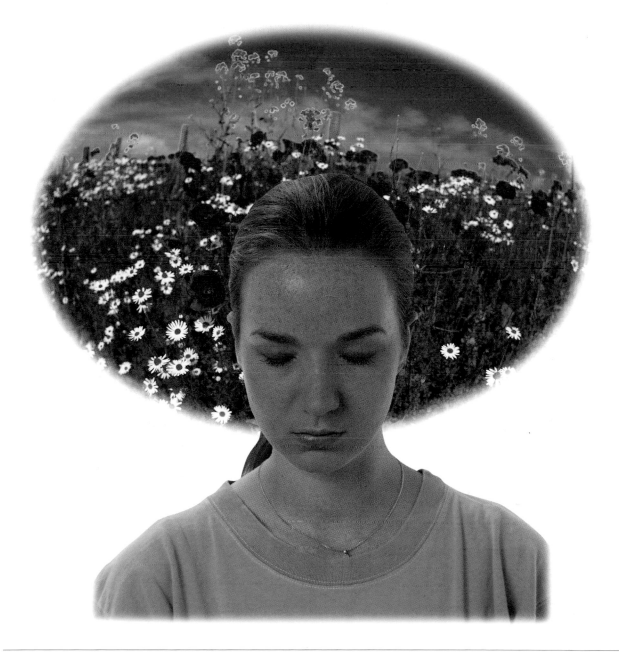

Basic Nutrition

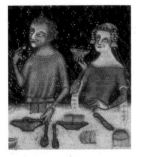

ABOVE *Interest in the relationship between food and health dates back centuries.*

THE STUDY OF FOOD *in relation to the physiological processes and well-being of the body goes back to antiquity. The science of nutrition incorporates both the study of diets and that of deficiency diseases caused by improper diet. It is no good balancing the body systems with reflexology if the wrong diet is causing further imbalances to the system.*

Nutrients essential for health include carbohydrates, fats, proteins, minerals, and vitamins. The body needs food for growth, repair of tissues, and energy. For the first two functions, you should include in your diet sufficient, but not an excess of, protein and fat, as these help cell renewal, the manufacture of body tissues, and vital circulating substances, such as enzymes (proteins that act as "biological catalysts" for reactions inside the body) and hormones. For energy, it is good to provide enough carbohydrates of the complex kind (such as vegetables and whole cereals), which are burned slowly to provide a continuous energy supply, rather than refined (such as white sugar), which is broken down too rapidly and soon leaves you short of energy again.

A healthy diet keeps your heart healthy. A good and varied diet would include plenty of fish (particularly oily fish) and some poultry, fresh vegetables and fruits, salads, wholegrain cereal products, and reduced-fat dairy products such as skimmed milk. This type of diet provides the necessary amino acids, which are the building blocks for creating new proteins. However, the body uses only limited amounts to build new cells and repair worn-out tissues; those that are in excess of the body's needs cannot be stored, and are broken down in the liver, forming a waste substance called urea, which is then excreted by the kidneys. In addition, a healthy diet should include plenty of vegetable fiber; this insures that waste products are passed out of the body regularly, which in turn protects you from any bowel disorders.

Liquids are equally important; you should drink at least six glasses

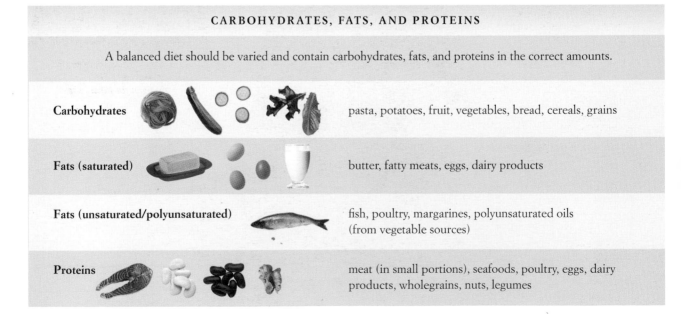

CARBOHYDRATES, FATS, AND PROTEINS

A balanced diet should be varied and contain carbohydrates, fats, and proteins in the correct amounts.

Carbohydrates		pasta, potatoes, fruit, vegetables, bread, cereals, grains
Fats (saturated)		butter, fatty meats, eggs, dairy products
Fats (unsaturated/polyunsaturated)		fish, poultry, margarines, polyunsaturated oils (from vegetable sources)
Proteins		meat (in small portions), seafoods, poultry, eggs, dairy products, wholegrains, nuts, legumes

of water daily. Water is seen as being of the utmost importance by all natural therapists, including reflexologists. Not only is our body composed mainly of water (approximately 73 percent), but this essential substance also aids both the transportation of nutrients and the elimination of toxic constituents (such as uric acid, a nitrogen-containing compound that, if it builds up in the tissue fluid, can lodge around the joints, causing inflammation of their lining). Water also helps lubricate the body at all levels, moisturizing the skin from the inside. We should also become aware of how much food we eat. If our diet includes more food than is needed to supply the body's immediate energy demands, then some of this surplus is stored by the liver for future use as a substance called glycogen, which can be quickly converted into glucose, the sugar that the body "burns" as its fuel; however, the rest becomes fat, stored around the abdomen or beneath the skin. There is some evidence, from animal experiments, that restricting the amount of food eaten can increase lifespan.

There are different diet recommendations for different groups of people. Eating less eggs, and offal such as liver and kidneys, is advisable for some people. For instance, kidney is very bad for gout sufferers. Most of us are able to cope with the waste product uric acid, and normally this is excreted in urine, but sometimes the body cannot cope and an excess of uric acid gradually develops.

JOINT INFLAMMATION

If the body's waste products are not flushed out of the system, they may cause joint inflammation.

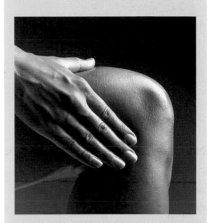

ABOVE *A build-up of toxins can cause tenderness, swelling, and pain in the joints.*

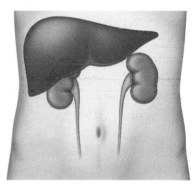

ABOVE *Excess food can be stored by the liver as glycogen for future use.*

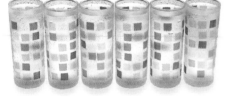

ABOVE *Try to drink at least six glasses of water every day.*

THIS WOMAN'S BODY CONTAINS APPROXIMATELY THIS MUCH WATER

RIGHT *Approximately 73 percent of our bodies is composed of water. It helps to transport nutrients.*

This lodges as crystals around the joints, causing gout, rheumatoid arthritis, and sometimes kidney disease. People who suffer from these problems need to cut down on their protein and try to eat more alkaline-forming foods (such as fresh fruit and vegetables), rather than acid-forming foods (such as dairy products).

In pregnancy, the expectant mother needs regular supplies of amino acids in her diet, along with enough calcium, iron, other minerals, and vitamins. It is these that build the proteins necessary for the developing baby for its tissue growth, calcium to aid the growth of bones, and the right amount of iron required for the blood – all necessary nutrients supplied in an adequate diet.

In general, everyone should try to avoid food containing chemical additives. This is much more difficult today, as chemicals are added to food at every stage. However, some of these chemicals can build up in the body and cause formation of toxins, adding to any toxic overload and counteracting the effect of the reflexology treatment. Chemical additives can also be a trigger for allergic reactions. Many people experience a very tender liver and kidney reflex during reflexology; this indicates a high level of toxins within the system, from medication or from an incorrect diet. So, the eliminative channels need to be stimulated to clear any toxic overload.

Nutrition is taken from the Latin word for nourish, "*nutritus*". However, nutrition is more than just nourishment, it is the actual process by which plants, animals, and humans take in nutrients and then absorb them in to their tissues.

Every cell in our body is dependent on nourishment. Once food has been digested and absorbed into the bloodstream, each cell then selects the constituents that are necessary for its continued health and growth. The system of physical and chemical changes within the body, the metabolism, is responsible for the production of energy, elimination of waste material

RIGHT *Gout is one of the most common forms of joint disease, especially in elderly men – affecting 16 men in every 1,000.*

RIGHT *A healthy diet is particularly vital for expectant women, as it will provide the required nutrients, both for the mother and the growing baby.*

PREGNANT WOMEN NEED THE CORRECT AMOUNT OF VITAMINS AND MINERALS IN THEIR DIET

BELOW *Gout sufferers should avoid too many dairy and offal products in their diet, such as cheese or liver.*

CHEESE

GOUT COMMONLY OCCURS AT THE BASE OF THE BIG TOE

BELOW *Pregnant women need calcium in their diet to build bones in their unborn baby.*

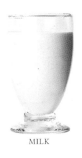

MILK

and growth, repair, and functioning of all body systems. Consequently, there is a fundamental relationship between the food that we eat and the efficiency of each cell. If we eat well, each cell performs properly, keeping our bodies in peak order. If, however, our diet is poor, our cells are unable to maintain themselves, the organs and tissues of the body become impaired and our health suffers.

Hippocrates (*c*.460–377 B.C.E.) was the first to note that ill health was often due to poor eating habits. Since then, physicians have studied our dietary requirements and concluded that certain foods can help prevent disease and others can aid the healing process. The Chinese have always placed great importance on the use of correct, health-building foods, and call this food therapy. Most Chinese medical books contain recipes that give specific methods of preparation for longevity and prevention of disease.

We are all responsible for our own health and well-being. An increased awareness of our dietary requirements will insure that our body receives the correct, essential nutrients in adequate amounts. Ignorance of our body's nutritional demands is just as hazardous as insatiable overeating.

The secret of a healthy diet is to eat only pure, natural foods, fruit, vegetables, and salad. Food is essential to life but do not assume that the more you eat, the more energy you will have. Energy and strength is totally unique to each individual; food merely enables us to make the best use of it.

FOOD ALLERGIES

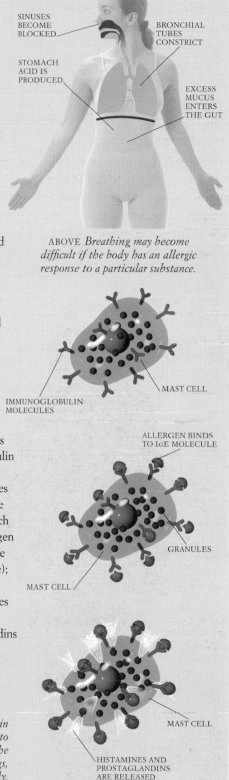

We know that in food allergies the body produces excess histamine (a protein); this hypersensitive response causes the body lining to swell to the degree that constriction of the bronchial (lung) tubes and even circulatory blockage can develop. In allergies such as asthma, hayfever, severe dermatitis (skin inflammation), or gastroenteritis (inflammation of the stomach and gut, or intestines), large amounts of mucus are produced in response to an irritant; the lungs, nose, and the sinuses then become clogged and excess mucus enters the gut. Diet here is very important; all dairy products should be limited as they are inclined to thicken the mucus, while fresh fruits and vegetables and spring water will help eliminate excess sticky mucus.

SINUSES BECOME BLOCKED

STOMACH ACID IS PRODUCED

BRONCHIAL TUBES CONSTRICT

EXCESS MUCUS ENTERS THE GUT

ABOVE *Breathing may become difficult if the body has an allergic response to a particular substance.*

The Allergic Response

Sometimes the immune system overreacts to seemingly harmless substances (allergens). In certain people, the immune system produces an antibody known as immunoglobulin E (IgE), which plays a prime part in allergic reaction. These IgE molecules cover the surface of mast cells. These molecules each have a receptor, which can interlock and bind with an allergen (a substance that when taken into the body, makes the body hypersensitive); this can come from pollen, feathers, fur, or dustmites. This causes granules inside the mast cell to release the inflammatory substances prostaglandins and histamine. It is these substances that trigger the allergic response.

MAST CELL

IMMUNOGLOBULIN MOLECULES

ALLERGEN BINDS TO IgE MOLECULE

GRANULES

MAST CELL

MAST CELL

HISTAMINES AND PROSTAGLANDINS ARE RELEASED

RIGHT *Mast cells are found in connective tissue adjacent to blood vessels and in the lymphatic system, skin, lungs, and other tissues of the body.*

Basic Techniques

BEFORE STARTING to work on specific areas, a number of general points need to be observed. The first step is to examine the person's foot, hand, or ear closely. This will allow you to see whether there are any abnormalities in the skin or detect sensitive areas, which may indicate imbalances that can cause an internal disorder, and help you decide where to concentrate your attention. Secondly, you should prepare for your treatment properly and collect together any articles you may need. Finally, you should be aware of the best holds and pressure techniques to employ for each body area.

FOOT AND HAND

There are three stages to examining the foot. The first is to note how the person walks, as this can indicate possible mechanical defects, and those arising from faulty footwear or bad posture. After this, you can examine the feet visually; any abnormalities in skin elasticity, texture, color, temperature, or humidity can all indicate an imbalance in your internal body functioning, and the presence of any skin conditions such as dermatitis, or infections such as ringworm or athlete's foot (both fungal), or verrucas (viral). The condition of nails can also be important, as changes in color, abnormal nail growth, or the presence of flecks, ridges, and white spots, can all indicate disorders. Finally, examination of the foot by touch allows you to assess the person's general pain threshold and enables you to check for ultrasensitive spots (these spots can be detected by palpation) that may indicate an imbalance in particular organs, or for marked insensitivity, which could indicate nerve damage. The hand should also be examined in a similar manner.

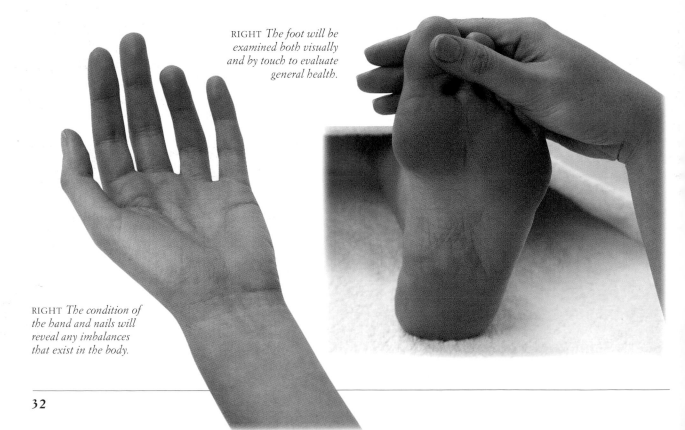

RIGHT *The foot will be examined both visually and by touch to evaluate general health.*

RIGHT *The condition of the hand and nails will reveal any imbalances that exist in the body.*

EAR

First, carefully examine the ear from top to bottom in a good light. Color is a good indication of general health; deep red areas can indicate a problem in the corresponding body area, and there may be pain and discomfort when pressure is applied to this area of the ear.

Secondly, note any blemishes, no matter how small. Check the corresponding ear for comparison. When any swelling or raised area is found, see if it is tender when pressed with a finger. Often, this area will feel puffy and tight, and again this indicates that there is a problem in the corresponding body area. Refer to the ear chart in Appendix One (*see p. 135*).

EXAMINING YOUR NAILS

- Ridges and fanning lines on nails, or excessively curved "hooked" growth, can indicate an overactive thyroid gland.
- Vertical ridges can indicate shock or trauma.
- Horizontal lines may indicate an overacid condition, respiratory problems, or trauma.
- Pitted nails may indicate a skin disorder, e.g., eczema or dermatitis.
- Spoon-shaped nails may mean an iron deficiency.
- White spots can indicate weak constitution, or trauma.
- Very white nails can mean a systemic disorder.
- Blue or purple nails may mean poor circulation.
- Slightly detached and yellow nails generally indicate an infection.

GENERAL POINTS FOR TREATMENT

- Find a comfortable place for the person to lie or sit (depending on the area being worked), and always use a support cushion for the legs or arms, or behind the head.
- Have all utensils to hand, such as wipes to clean hands, as well as clean towels, cotton buds to apply direct pressure on ear points, fingers, or thumbs. For ear and face treatment, offer a hairband if the person has long hair.

- Ask the person to remove his or her rings or earrings, as appropriate, and remove your own rings.
- Keep your nails clipped to avoid hurting the person when applying pressure.
- Remember each individual's pain threshold may differ, so you must be able to adapt your pressure; to begin with, less is often better.

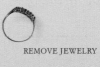

REMOVE JEWELRY

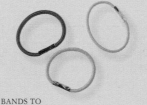

BANDS TO
RESTRAIN HAIR

COTTON BUDS
FOR APPLYING
PRESSURE

ABOVE *Before a treatment, make sure you have everything you need at hand; the patient should remove their jewelry.*

BELOW *The practitioner will examine the ear all over for swellings or blemishes.*

Supporting and Holding Techniques

DIFFERENT SUPPORT AND HOLDING TECHNIQUES *may be used so that the area being worked upon is held most effectively. This allows you to achieve the optimum comfort for you and your patient. Gently, but firmly, support the patient's hand or foot with your hand, forming a crutch. Also, make sure that you never pull the patient's skin taut; instead, let the foot or hand being held fall naturally, so that there is no tension created within it.*

SHAKING HANDS
The standard hold when working on the hands is the "shaking hands" position.

GRIP FOR THE LOWER FOOT
When you are working the area of the foot below the waistline, allow the person's heel to rest in the palm of your supporting hand. Your thumb should rest on the notch just below the person's big toe, as this stops the foot splaying out.

STANDARD FOOT HOLD
If you are working the front area of the foot (above the waistline), then hold it from above, with the web of your hand touching the side of the foot, your four fingers on the top of the foot, and your thumb pressing lightly on the ball of the foot. Gently stretch the top of the foot or the back of the hand so that the toes are not bent back away from you.

REST HEEL IN HAND

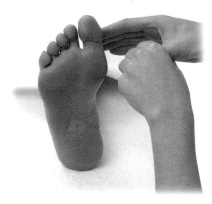

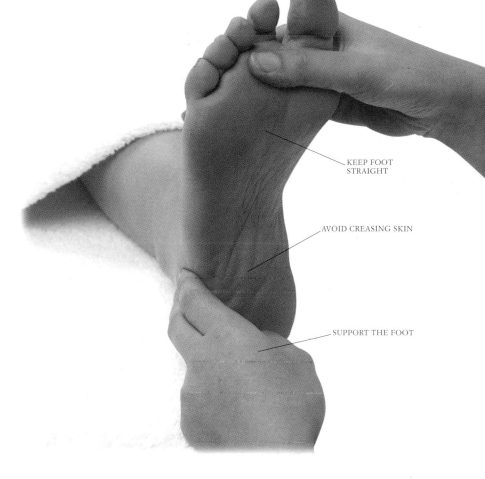

KEEP FOOT
STRAIGHT

AVOID CREASING SKIN

SUPPORT THE FOOT

WORKING THE DORSAL SURFACE

To work the top of the foot (the dorsal surface), make a fist of your support hand. Place the thumb of your working hand in between the thumb and forefinger of your support hand; this allows a pincer action. For the back of the hand, link your right thumb in with the person's right thumb, supporting the whole hand in your palm.

SUPPORT USING FLAT OF HAND

You can also support the foot using the flat of your hand, either the palm or the back.

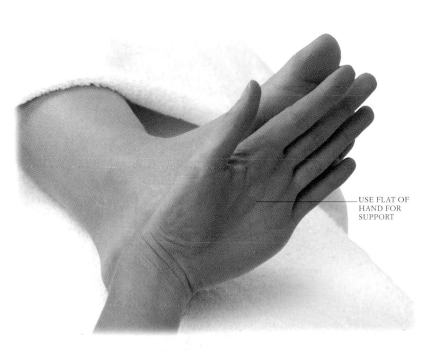

USE FLAT OF
HAND FOR
SUPPORT

WORKING THE MEDIAL OR LATERAL EDGE

When working the inside (medial) or outside (lateral) edge of the foot or hand, keep it as straight as possible (vertical for the foot, and horizontal for the hand). This allows you to avoid creasing the skin on the heel or pad at the base of the palm, which hinders movement. Use a support hold (see p. 34) and work as follows: to work the inner edge, support the person's left foot with your right hand and work with your left; for the outer edge you will need to change hands so that your left hand supports this foot and your right hand does the work (and so on).

Pressure Techniques

THERE ARE MANY *different ways of applying pressure to the skin. In some of these, the pressure is applied and then released; in others, the pressure is maintained as the hands are moved, as in massage. In different areas, it is appropriate to apply pressure with the thumb, fingers, knuckles, or palms.*

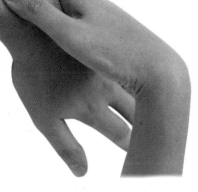

THUMB PRESSURE

ALTERNATING THUMB OR FINGER PRESSURE

This is a very precise technique for working particular reflex points. In this technique, the thumb (or finger) is used to apply palpation or alternating pressure to a point for a moment or so. The pressure is then released (although your thumb maintains contact with the person's skin), the thumb is moved to the next point, and the pressure is applied once more.

ROTATING THUMB, FINGER, OR KNUCKLE PRESSURE

Use the pad of the thumb so that your nail doesn't dig into the person's skin. Press firmly into the reflex point and, keeping this pressure constant, make two or three small clockwise or counterclockwise rotations around the point. Then release the pressure and move your thumb to the next point, as in the alternating pressure technique. (You can also perform this technique by using the index and middle fingers or the knuckle.)

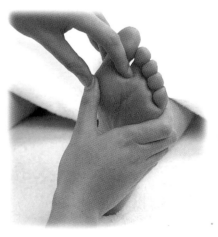

PRESS FIRMLY

USE PAD OF THUMB

ROTATING THUMB PRESSURE

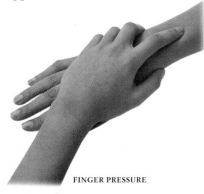

FINGER PRESSURE

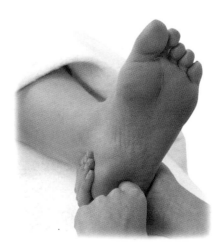

ROTATING KNUCKLE PRESSURE

ROTATING FINGER PRESSURE

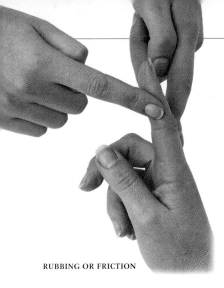

RUBBING OR FRICTION

RUBBING OR FRICTION

Rubbing creates a friction effect and can therefore be used to warm and relax the body area to be worked. It can be used to massage each of the fingers or toes separately. Using the thumb on one side of the digit and the index finger on the other in a pincer hold, rub gently, moving the thumb and first finger in opposite directions. You can also use your two palms to rub the edges of the foot (*refer to side friction technique, p. 39*).

KNEADING

Kneading is useful on areas where the skin is insensitive or thick and tough (such as the heel), and where more pressure is needed for stimulation. Use your knuckles to make a fist. Either use a slightly circular action as if you were kneading dough, kneading the whole foot, or push and squeeze with the supporting hand in a to-and-fro motion (*refer to kneading and knuckling, pp. 39 and 42*).

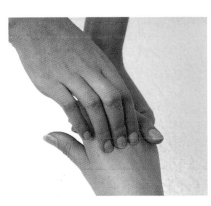

WALKING ON HANDS (DORSAL)

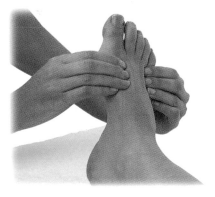

WALKING ON FEET (DORSAL)

WALKING

Walking can be used to apply gentle pressure to a large area, (this is both relaxing and therapeutic) such as the top (dorsal) surface of the hand or foot. It may be done with one or both hands. The fist of the supporting hand should be placed on the palm or sole to support it (use the thumbs if both hands are working). Then, using one, two, or three fingers (whichever is most comfortable) in an alternating movement, finger-walk down or across the foot or hand. Start either at the toes or the fingers and then work toward the ankle or wrist, or start at the side and meet at the top of the dorsal surface (*see p. 41*).

KNEADING WITH KNUCKLE

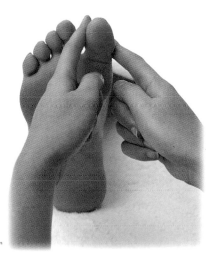

RUBBING OR FRICTION

USE CIRCULAR ACTIONS AS IF KNEADING DOUGH

MAKE A FIST WITH YOUR KNUCKLES

Preliminary Relaxation Sequence

THE RELAXATION TECHNIQUES *are aimed at loosening muscular tension in the body and the part being worked on. They are recommended for use before commencing specific treatment. They can be used in any order and repeated whenever necessary. You can also use them at points throughout the treatment session, some being used to begin working certain areas. These basic procedures are suitable for both the hands and feet.*

SIDE TO SIDE RELAXATION

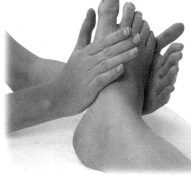

SIDE TO SIDE RELAXATION
Place your hands either side of the ball of the foot, then move the foot alternately backward and forward between them. This loosens the upper part of the body, alleviating stiff shoulders and relaxing the respiratory tract. On the hands, this is done with the person's palm facing you; slot your thumbs in between the thumb and little finger.

SIDE TO SIDE RELAXATION ON HANDS

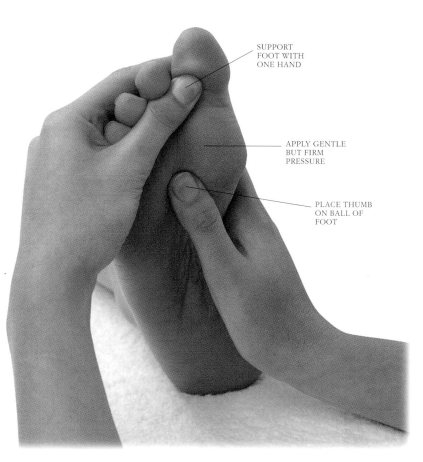

SUPPORT FOOT WITH ONE HAND

APPLY GENTLE BUT FIRM PRESSURE

PLACE THUMB ON BALL OF FOOT

DIAPHRAGM RELAXATION

DIAPHRAGM RELAXATION
This also aids breathing. Place your thumb of the working hand on the ball of the foot at the inner (medial) edge and apply gentle but firm pressure; at the same time support with the other hand (see support hold, p. 34). *Again this can be done on the hands, but always support from the little-finger side and work across the base of the finger pads, repeating several times.*

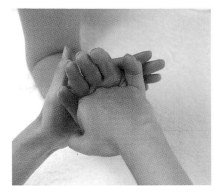

KNEADING HANDS

MOLDING THE FOOT OR HAND

Both palms working together, place one on the top surface and one on the palm or sole. Working from the outside (lateral) edge (to insure that not too much pressure is applied to the great toe or thumb joint), mold as if you were rolling dough in your hands. This relaxes the rib cage area, lungs/chest, heart, and shoulders.

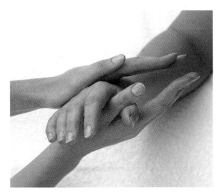

MOLDING THE HANDS

KNEADING THE BASE OF THE TOES OR FINGERS

Make a fist with your palm, your knuckles in line with the base of the toes on the sole of the foot and the support hand on the top surface (your index finger in line with the base of the toes). Push with your knuckle and squeeze with your support hand alternately. This relaxes the shoulder girdle, as well as aiding the lung and chest area. Use your right hand to the right foot, and left hand to left foot, working from the outside (lateral) edge to insure no undue pressure is put on the great toe joint. This can also be done on the hands to knead the bones at the base of the fingers, which are known as the metacarpals (see p. 45).

PLACE ONE HAND ON TOP SURFACE

MOLD AS IF ROLLING DOUGH

PLACE OTHER HAND ON SOLE

MOLDING THE FOOT

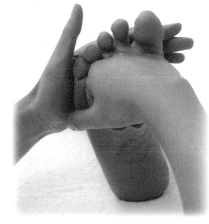

KNEADING FEET

SIDE FRICTION

Both palms are used, on the inside and outside edges of the foot or hand. Slide your hands up and down the surface alternately. Do this to warm the limb, and to relieve stress or tension quickly.

USE PALMS ON EDGE OF FEET

SLIDE HANDS UP AND DOWN THE FOOT

SIDE FRICTION

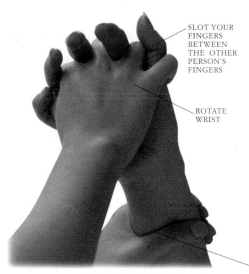

SLOT YOUR
FINGERS
BETWEEN
THE OTHER
PERSON'S
FINGERS

ROTATE
WRIST

SUPPORT WRIST

WRIST ROTATION

ACHILLES TENDON STRETCH

Using the same hold as for ankle rotation, stretch the whole foot backward and forward. This relaxes the calf muscles and the arches of the foot and, because the Achilles tendon is joined to the heel, will also affect the wrists, ankles, pelvic areas, and hips. To stretch the tendons of the arm, use the same hold as in the wrist rotation, but this time flexing and extending the wrist.

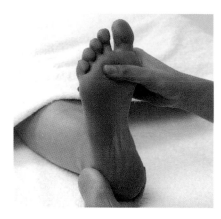

STRETCH THE FOOT BACKWARD

ANKLE AND WRIST ROTATION

When working the feet, gently rotate the ankle, supporting the heel with one hand, your thumb pointing toward the little toe, and the other hand supporting the great toe joint. Rotate in both directions several times. When working the hands, slot your fingers between the other person's fingers, support from the wrist, and rotate the wrist both ways.

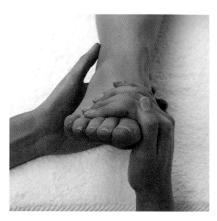

STRETCH THE FOOT FORWARD

ANKLE ROTATION

SUPPORTING THE
FOOT, GENTLY
ROTATE THE ANKLE
IN A CIRCULAR
MOTION IN EACH
DIRECTION

SUPPORT
FOOT

ROTATE EACH
FINGER BOTH WAYS

SUPPORT
PALM OF
HAND

**FINGER STRETCHING
AND ROTATION**

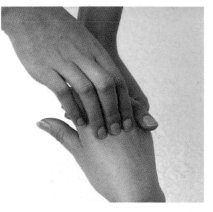

WALKING ON HANDS (DORSAL)

TOE AND FINGER STRETCHING AND ROTATION

Gently stretch and rotate each toe and finger both ways. You can support the ball of the foot, or the palm of the hand if you wish.

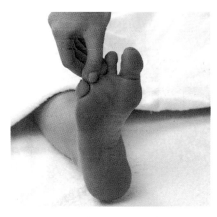

TOE STRETCHING AND ROTATION

RIBCAGE TECHNIQUE

Place your thumbs on the palm of the hand or the sole of the foot, tuck up the first three fingers of each of your hands and work them in an alternating movement up from the sides until they almost meet on the center line of the top (dorsal) surface (be careful not to pinch the last little bit of skin). Repeat this several times, working gradually up the foot or hand to the waistline. This stimulates the lungs, chest/breast area, and shoulder girdle.

WALKING DOWN

This relaxes the whole torso. Using three fingers, with your fist supporting on the sole or palm, work down to the waist area (the line from the base of the web between the thumb and index finger) on the top (dorsal) surface.

ABDOMINAL WALKING

Using the same hold as for ribcage technique left, finger-walk (see p. 37) in slight diagonal lines on the top surface of the foot. This relaxes the abdominal wall, stimulating the abdominal and pelvic muscles, and aids the lower back.

RIBCAGE TECHNIQUE

PLACE
THUMBS
ON SOLES
OF FEET

WORK HANDS UP
FROM THE SIDES
TO THE CENTER

CAUTION

Insure that you do this gently, particularly with an arthritis sufferer, so that you do not cause pain or further damage to a joint. Leave it out if there are any severe health problems that contraindicate its use.

WRIST LOOSENING

PLACE PAD IN WRIST DEPRESSION

MOVE HANDS ALTERNATELY

HACKING

KNUCKLING THE FOOT OR HAND
Using a loose, two-finger knuckle (index and big finger), sweep down the foot or hand in vertical strips. If the knuckles are used when working a reflex, always use the inner (medial) edge of your index finger in a circular movement; this gives light friction to the area. (See knuckling of spine.)

ANKLE AND WRIST LOOSENING
Place the pad at the base of your thumb in the depression of the person's heel or wrist area and move the foot or hand from side to side. This should not be painful; do not apply pressure on the ankle or wrist bone, or shake the foot or hand from side to side.

HACKING
This is better done on the feet and toes. Rhythmically apply a sideways light, brisk stroke up and down the sole of the foot. Use your fingers (not the heel of your hand) on the little-finger side of the hand.

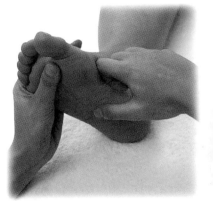

KNUCKLING ON SPINE REFLEX

ANKLE LOOSENING

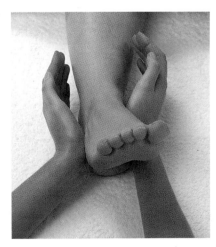

KNUCKLING

STROKE THE PALM OF THE HAND

USE A LOOSE TWO-FINGER KNUCKLE

EFFECTS OF RELAXATION TECHNIQUES

These relaxation techniques help to stimulate local circulation, often achieving a pain relieving effect in the corresponding body part and therefore aiding muscular tension.

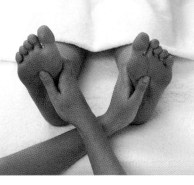

SOLAR PLEXUS ROTATION

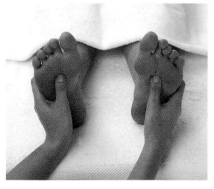

SOLAR PLEXUS RELAXATION

SOLAR PLEXUS ROTATION (FEET ONLY)

Cross your hands, then put your thumbs on the reflex points just behind the ball of the foot. Rotate your thumbs in an inward direction three times. (This is easier to do after you have applied a little cream and have massaged the lower leg and foot at the end of the treatment.)

SOLAR PLEXUS RELAXATION (FEET ONLY)

Place both thumbs on the same points as solar plexus rotation. Apply firm, unmoving pressure as the person takes a breath. Repeat this three times.

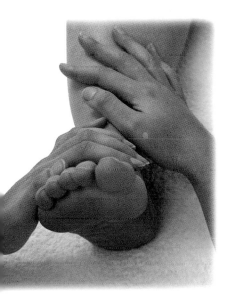

SWEEPING STROKES

SWEEPING STROKES

These can be applied over the whole foot or hand rhythmically. This increases blood flow and generally disperses any excess fluid, reducing swelling (edema). Always work toward the heart.

PUMMELING

Using a closed fist and the heel of your hand, strike the heel or the base pad of the hand several times. This softens the solid, firm tissue, and aids the lower back.

PUMMELING

USE CLOSED
FIST

STRIKE BASE
OF HAND
SEVERAL
TIMES

Reflexology of the Feet and Hands

THIS PART OF THE BOOK *reviews each of the body systems in turn and locates the reflex zones on the feet and hands. It then shows how both the foot and the hand may be worked according to the body area or organ system they correspond to. Although the illustrations show working in one direction only, all areas may also be worked in the opposite direction in order to maximize stimulation to that area. Each sequence here can be regarded either as a preventative treatment to maintain the health of the body system, or as a specific therapy to aid an imbalance. Common disorders for each system are not listed here, however, as they are covered later.*

ABOVE *Hands and feet are both used in reflexology treatment.*

The feet are the most widely used site for reflexology treatment. They are the foundation of our body and support the weight of the whole skeleton, producing movement and acting as effective shock absorbers. However, just like any building or superstructure, if the underpinning is faulty, then serious defects may appear later. Poor biomechanics of the feet, whether caused by hereditary defects, bad habits resulting from poor choice of footwear, incorrect posture, or as an effect of falls and other accidents, ultimately are reflected in spinal distortions and are frequently accompanied by nerve irritations as high as the head and imbalances in body systems.

RIGHT *The feet are the most common part of the body worked on by reflexologists.*

Although the feet are the usual choice for reflexologists, the hands are also used in acupressure and shiatsu treatment, and acupuncture is widely used on the hands in China. A full reflexology treatment can be given to the hands instead of the feet as there is less toxin release. There are also additional reflex points on the hands that can help a variety of disorders as extra target reflexes for specific problems, and as a convenient site for self-treatment and first aid.

THE BODY SYSTEMS AND THE REFLEX POINTS

The body systems do not function in isolation, but are interdependent and also rely on the finely tuned balance of every organ within that system. Each of the body systems is represented on particular areas of the foot and hand. In general, however, as you go down the body there is a progression of reflex areas from the tips of the digits to the heel of the foot or base of the hand, so the brain and head reflex areas are found around the digits, the chest and thorax areas at the front of the foot and hand, the abdominal regions in the middle, and the reproductive organs of the lower trunk and the pelvis at the rear of the foot and the base of the hand.

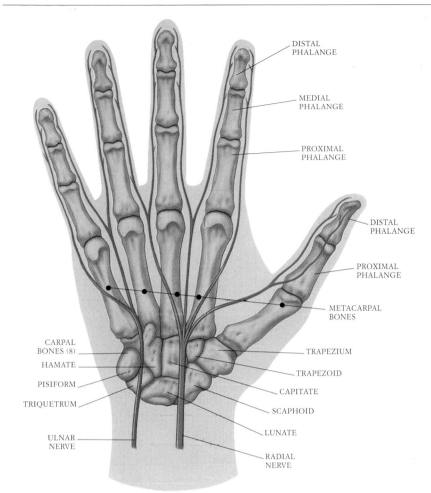

DISTAL
PHALANGE

MEDIAL
PHALANGE

PROXIMAL
PHALANGE

DISTAL
PHALANGE

PROXIMAL
PHALANGE

METACARPAL
BONES

CARPAL
BONES (8)

HAMATE

PISIFORM

TRIQUETRUM

ULNAR
NERVE

TRAPEZIUM

TRAPEZOID

CAPITATE

SCAPHOID

LUNATE

RADIAL
NERVE

STRUCTURE OF THE FOOT AND HAND

The foot and the hand have a very similar structure. This is understandable if you remember that at some time in their evolution all bipedal animals had ancestors that walked on all fours. The structure of the foot and hand can each be divided into three main sections: the bones making up the digits (thumbs, fingers, toes), which are scientifically termed the phalanges; the bones making up the hand and the foot, which are termed the metacarpals and the metatarsals, respectively; and the bones making up the wrist and the hindfoot/ankle, which are termed the carpals and tarsals, respectively. There is a rich supply of nerve endings in the hands and feet, giving them an amazing sensitivity.

ABOVE AND BELOW *The hands and feet can both be divided into three sections and are very similar in construction.*

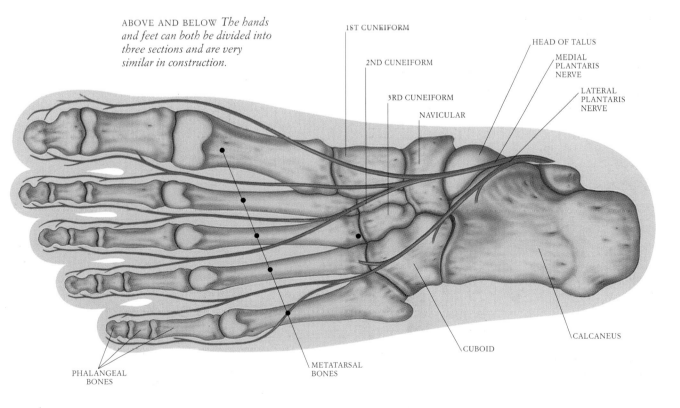

1ST CUNEIFORM

2ND CUNEIFORM

3RD CUNEIFORM

NAVICULAR

HEAD OF TALUS

MEDIAL
PLANTARIS
NERVE

LATERAL
PLANTARIS
NERVE

PHALANGEAL
BONES

METATARSAL
BONES

CUBOID

CALCANEUS

Head-related Areas

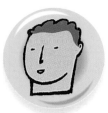

ABOVE *The head acts as the body's general command center.*

HEAD-RELATED AREAS *include the reflexes for the brain, eyes, ears, facial area, nose, sinuses, mouth, jaw, the trigeminal nerve running to them, the neck and muscles to the neck and shoulder. Reflexology treatment can help clear mild infections, stimulate the sensory organs, and also act as a painkiller.*

The brain is a vastly complex coordination and command center, receiving and transmitting electrical and chemical impulses from and to regions of the body. The head area also includes a number of specialized sensory organs – the eyes, ears, nose, and tongue.

BELOW *The head area contains specialized sensory organs.*

The reflexes for the head-related areas are found on the upper and lower surfaces of the toes and fingers. Treat them by working all the digits on feet or hands in turn. When working here, imagine that you are working on a bed of pins, and each pin in turn must be pressed down – this is how small the alternating steps must be. Treatment can relieve minor infections, clearing excess mucus so that it does not enter the sinuses or middle ear via the eustachian tube (which connects the middle ear to the throat). It can stimulate the organs of balance, hearing, sight, and smell. It can also act as an analgesic, for example in the case of toothache or trigeminal neuralgia (nerve inflammation, which causes jaw or facial pain).

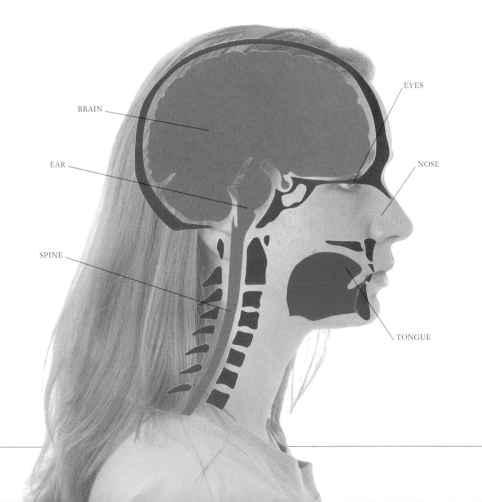

BRAIN

EYES

EAR

NOSE

SPINE

TONGUE

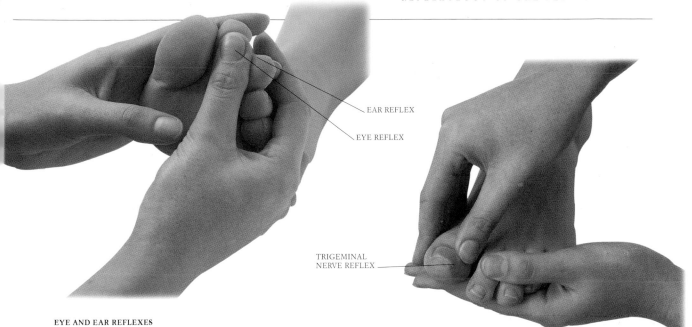

EAR REFLEX

EYE REFLEX

TRIGEMINAL
NERVE REFLEX

EYE AND EAR REFLEXES

THE EYE AND EAR REFLEXES
*These are on the distal joints at the
tips of the digits (the former are on
the second and third digits, the latter
on the third and fourth). Rotate or
palpate these several times.*

THE FACIAL AREA AND
TEETH REFLEXES
*These reflexes are found on the
dorsal surfaces of all the toes
and fingers.*

THE TRIGEMINAL NERVE REFLEX
*This is on the outside (lateral) edge
of the thumb or great toe.*

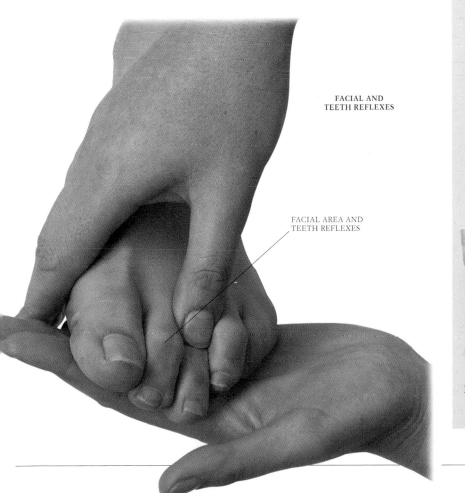

FACIAL AND
TEETH REFLEXES

FACIAL AREA AND
TEETH REFLEXES

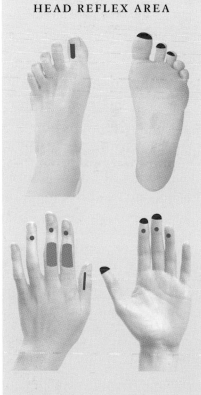

HEAD REFLEX AREA

Individual reflex points are detailed on the
charts in Appendix One (pp.130–35).

The Respiratory System

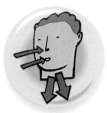

ABOVE *The respiratory system provides fresh oxygen to our blood.*

THE RESPIRATORY SYSTEM *encompasses the sinuses and nose, the organs of the chest cavity involved in breathing, including the lungs and diaphragm, and the connecting passageways – the pharynx (throat), larynx (voicebox), trachea (windpipe), and bronchial tubes. Reflexology treatment will help breathing as well as clear congestions and calm inflammation.*

The reflexes to the respiratory areas are at the front of the foot and hand, on both upper and lower surfaces, extending to the diaphragm line (*see p. 8*). The reflexes to the heart are covered under the circulatory system (*see pp. 60–61*). Treatment of this area clears congestion in the mucus-producing sinus and nasal cavities, calms inflammation, and aids breathing. It can also reduce excessive mucus production; although we need mucus to trap particles entering the respiratory tract, if the hair fronds (cilia) here do not function properly, then the mucus-secreting cells enlarge and increase production to protect these passageways; they then become a breeding ground for bacteria.

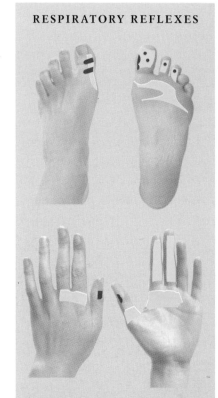

RESPIRATORY REFLEXES

Individual reflex points are detailed on the charts in Appendix One (pp.130–35).

RIGHT *The respiratory system provides oxygen to the blood as well as removing carbon dioxide from the body.*

NASAL CAVITY

LARYNX

LUNGS

TRACHEA

DIAPHRAGM

TREATMENT AIMS

Work on these reflexes aims to facilitate the whole breathing process, aiding the diaphragm and the intercostal muscles.

LUNG AREA

Commence by working the lung area on the pads below the first to fourth toes and the first to third fingers. Work both the area between the joints and also on the joints themselves.

Start working in vertical strips, then repeat in horizontal strips, covering the whole area from the diaphragm line to the bases of the digits across the whole width of the hand or foot (even though the lungs finish on the third zone, if you do this you also cover the shoulder region). Use your thumbs on the sole or palm area and your index fingers on the top (dorsal) surfaces.

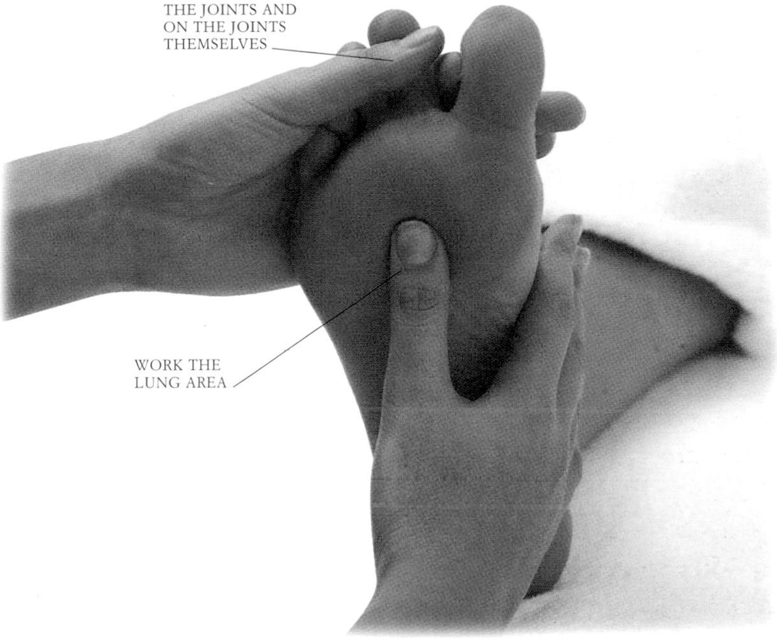

WORK BETWEEN THE JOINTS AND ON THE JOINTS THEMSELVES

WORK THE LUNG AREA

LUNG REFLEXES

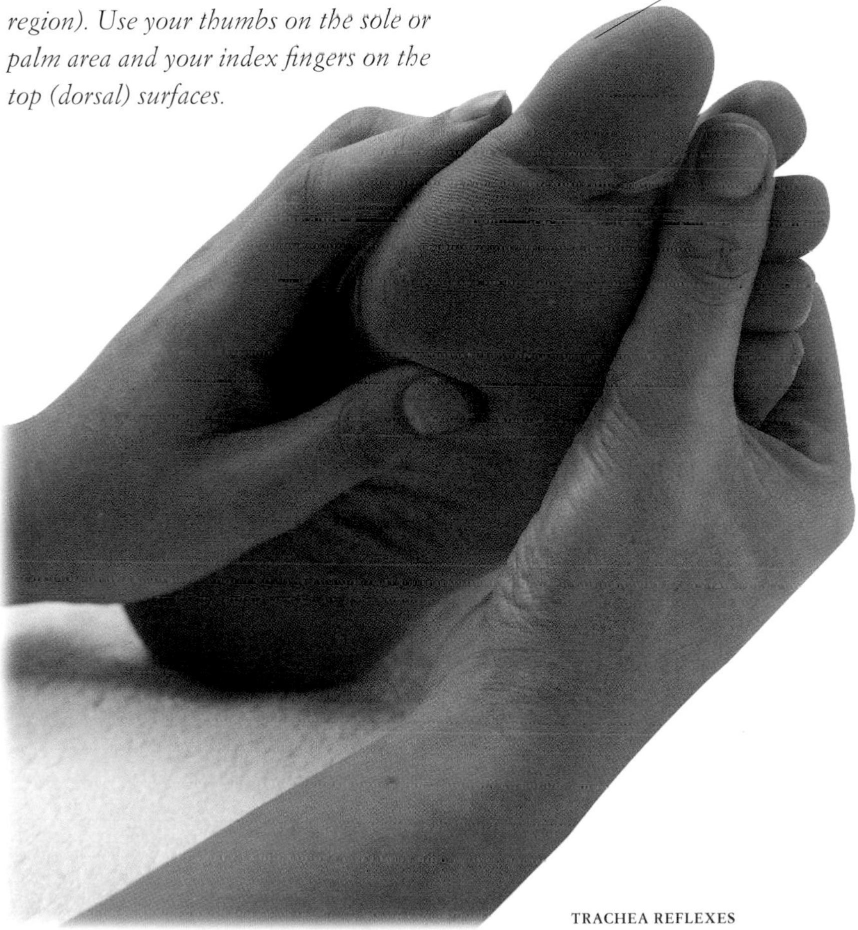

TRACHEA REFLEX

THE TRACHEA REFLEX
This is on the inner (medial) edge of the great toe or thumb.

THE DIAPHRAGM REFLEX
This is in between the ball of the foot and the arch.

TRACHEA REFLEXES

The Endocrine System

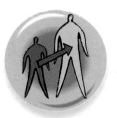

ABOVE *Hormones in the brain regulate growth patterns.*

THE ENDOCRINE SYSTEM *includes all the endocrine glands; this type of gland produces hormones, which are released directly into the bloodstream to circulate around the body. Hormones are chemicals that are released into the blood and balance the levels of important blood compounds, such as sugars and salts, and regulate processes such as growth, reproduction, and responses to stress.*

In the brain, the hypothalamus produces hormones that regulate growth and many unconscious bodily activities – e.g., blood pressure, heart rate, urine output and peristalsis (*see The Digestive System, pp. 52–53*), and body rhythms such as the female menstrual cycle; it also controls the secretions of the pituitary gland, which oversees the hormone production of a number of other glands. The hypothalamus is also related to our emotional activity. The light-sensitive pineal gland in the midbrain is involved in both daily and seasonal body cycles, (including our sleep cycles – *see pp. 22–23*), through variations in its production of the hormones melatonin and serotonin. The thyroid gland in the throat controls our basal metabolic rate, speeding up or slowing down all our body processes. There is a complex connection between the thyroid and the nervous system in the regulation of metabolism, as the thyroid hormones affect the sensitivity of the frontal (anterior) lobe of the pituitary gland. The

parathyroid glands, lying behind the thyroid, are responsible for control of our calcium and phosphate levels. The paired adrenal glands are triangular-shaped organs that sit on top of the kidneys. These important glands not only influence our carbohydrate metabolism, but they also affect the immunological response. They produce hormones that reduce inflammation (as they are naturally occurring steroids), suppress allergic reactions, balance our sugar, mineral, and water levels, and prepare the body for fight or flight.

The reflexes to the endocrine areas lie on the lower surfaces of the foot and hand in both the frontal (for head and neck glands) and middle (for mid-body glands) areas, and also just below the digits on the top (dorsal) surface (thyroids and parathyroids). Treatment seems to stabilize glandular activity so that hormonal levels remain in optimal balance. The following endocrine organs are covered under other systems: the pancreas, which is an organ producing both hormones regulating blood sugar levels and digestive enzymes (*see Digestive System, pp. 52–53*) and the paired ovaries/testes (*see Reproductive System, pp. 56–57*).

PITUITARY GLAND

THYROID GLAND

ADRENAL GLANDS

PANCREAS

LEFT *The endocrine glands release hormones, which circulate in the blood and other bodily fluids.*

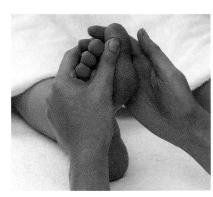

PITUITARY REFLEX

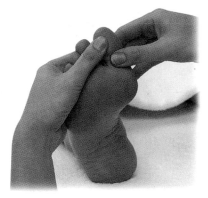

THYROID AND PARATHYROID REFLEXES

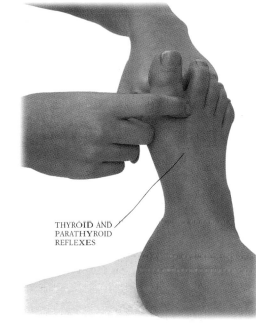

THYROID AND
PARATHYROID
REFLEXES

THYROID AND PARATHYROID REFLEXES

THE HYPOTHALAMUS, PITUITARY, AND PINEAL GLAND REFLEXES

These are found within the brain reflex on the great toe or thumb (see Head-related areas, pp. 46–47). We can give them an extra workout by applying extra pressure on the center of the pad of the thumb or great toe.

THE THYROID AND PARATHYROID GLAND REFLEXES

These are on the bases of the first three toes and thumb or fingers on both surfaces. This area can be worked both ways, using thumbs or index fingers.

THE ADRENAL GLAND REFLEX

This should be stimulated whenever an allergy is present and for all the inflammatory problems, helping many joint disorders, relieving pain, and reducing swelling.

STIMULATE THE
ADRENAL GLAND FOR
INFLAMMATORY PROBLEMS

ADRENAL REFLEX

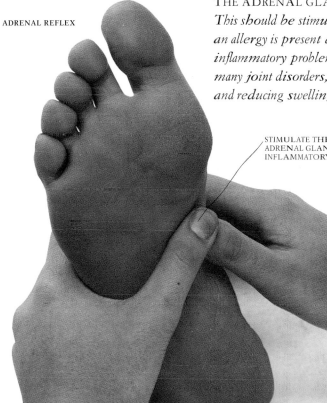

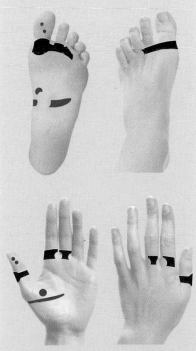

ENDOCRINE REFLEXES

Individual reflex points are detailed on the charts in Appendix One (pp.130–35).

The Digestive System

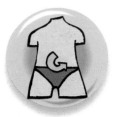

ABOVE *The digestive system is easily upset, often due to stress.*

THE DIGESTIVE SYSTEM *includes all the organs (stomach, liver, gallbladder, duodenum, and pancreas) and associated tracts, from the mouth to the anus, involved in the complicated process of digestion. In digestion, large, complex chemicals are broken down so that the body can absorb and use them for energy and other vital processes.*

The digestive process involves both chemical breakdown, by liver bile, stomach acid, and enzymes produced by several organs, and mechanical action, by the teeth and the intestinal muscles. Chemical breakdown begins in the mouth; saliva contains a starch-digesting enzyme. Broken-up food passes first into the stomach, where stomach acid breaks down proteins, then into the duodenum, which continues this breakdown and also secretes enzymes for carbohydrate and fat digestion. This process is aided by the pancreas, which secretes enzymes into the digestive tract for protein, carbohydrate, and fat digestion. The liver produces bile, a substance that helps in fat absorption (this is stored in the gallbladder); it also carries out important steps in the metabolism of carbohydrates,

fats, and proteins. Finally, it has an important detoxifying role, responding to any substance that may be poisonous to the system, whether ingested or formed by excess buildup of metabolic products or hormones.

The reflexes to the digestive system lie on the lower surface (sole or palm) of the foot and hand, in the middle and hind areas. Treatment encourages production of the digestive juices, aiding absorption of nutrients, and stimulates peristalsis, the rhythmic, "wormlike" process of contraction of intestinal and bowel muscles that propels food along the tract and mixes it with digestive hormones. The intestinal tract is particularly prone to abnormal functioning, often in response to stress. This can be much alleviated by reflexology.

RIGHT *The digestive system ingests, stores, and digests food. It also eliminates waste from the body.*

ESOPHAGUS

LIVER

STOMACH

SMALL INTESTINE

LARGE INTESTINE

RECTUM

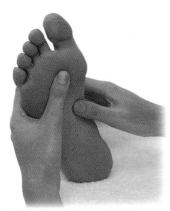

LIVER/GALLBLADDER REFLEXES

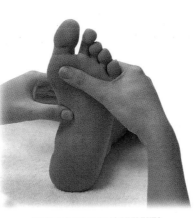

STOMACH/PANCREAS REFLEXES

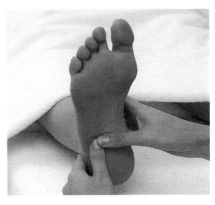

ILEOCECAL VALVE

LIVER/GALLBLADDER REFLEXES
These are in the middle of the sole and palm of the right foot and hand, between the waistline and the diaphragm line, from the first to the fourth zones. On the left foot and hand, the liver reflex is in the first zone only.

STOMACH/PANCREAS REFLEXES
These are worked on the left foot and hand in the same general area. The pancreas extends to the third zone just above the waistline. This area can be worked in diagonal strips or in horizontal strips, going both ways.

Four reflexes need extra attention:
(i) First, the reflex to the ileocecal valve, on the outside edge of the right foot and hand in line with the bladder and rectum; this valve controls movement between the small and large intestine.
(ii) The bends in the large intestine known as the hepatic (liver) and
(iii) splenic flexures are also important; both are on the waistline, the first on the right side under the liver reflex, and the second on the left side under the spleen reflex.
(iv) The sigmoid colon also needs extra pressure. This reflex is only on the left foot or hand.

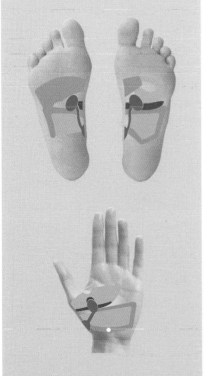

DIGESTIVE REFLEXES

Individual reflex points are detailed on the charts in Appendix One (pp.130–35).

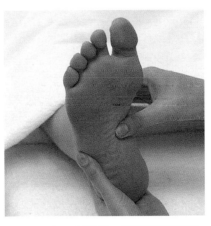

INTESTINAL REFLEX (II) – HEPATIC FLEXURE

THE INTESTINAL AREA
This area, from the waist down to the pelvic area, can be covered in horizontal strips, working both ways.

Apply firm pressure with the thumb on all these points. Finish with abdominal walking to relax the whole area (see p. 41).

SPLENIC
FLEXURE

SIGMOID COLON REFLEX

APPLY PRESSURE
WITH THUMB

INTESTINAL
REFLEX

The Urinary System

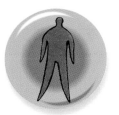

ABOVE *The urinary system regulates fluids in the body, which is made up of 73% water.*

THE URINARY SYSTEM *is the main excretory system of the body (others include the skin and the lungs). It includes the two kidneys (which act as a filtration unit, producing the liquid called urine), the ureter tubes, the bladder, and the urethra.*

The function of the urinary system is to remove from the body any waste metabolic products, some of which will become noxious if allowed to build up within the body tissues. It is a filtration system that also selectively reabsorbs the maximum of useful compounds, including vital salts and water, back into the body before the resultant liquid urine containing waste products is excreted from the urethra. The kidneys filter and clean approximately 25 percent of the blood supply at every single heartbeat, and continuously regulate the content of the urine, specifically the electrolyte and acid balance. The liquid that is excreted is largely a solution of nitrogenous waste from metabolized hormones and other proteins. The ureters are tubes carrying urine from the kidneys to the bladder. The bladder stores the urine until it fills and then passes it out of the body down the urethra. The urethra is the tube carrying urine from the bladder to the outside of the body.

The kidneys also produce a hormone in response to low oxygen levels that stimulates red blood cell production. The adrenal glands sited on top of the kidneys secrete, amongst other things, hormones regulating the body's salt water balance; they are covered under the Endocrine System (*see pp. 50–51*).

The reflexes to the urinary areas lie in the middle of the lower sole/palm and the inner (medial) surfaces of the foot and hand. Treatment is aimed at normalizing nerve signals to the bladder so that normal bladder action occurs. Treatment can help slight inflammation and balance uric acid levels in cases of repeated infections.

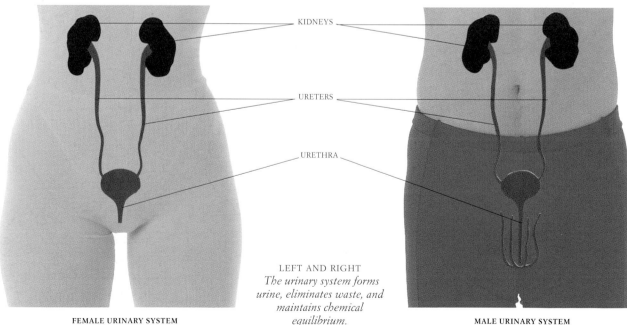

KIDNEYS

URETERS

URETHRA

FEMALE URINARY SYSTEM

LEFT AND RIGHT
The urinary system forms urine, eliminates waste, and maintains chemical equilibrium.

MALE URINARY SYSTEM

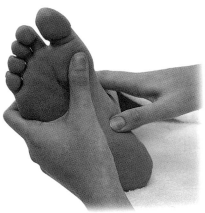

BLADDER REFLEX

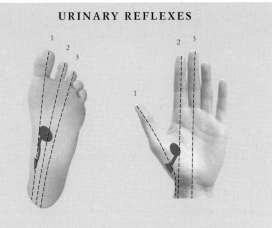

URINARY REFLEXES

Individual reflex points are detailed on the charts in Appendix One (pp.130–35).

BLADDER/URETHRA REFLEX

This is easy to find, as it lies on the inner (medial) edge of the foot and below and slightly in front of the ankle, on the raised padded area. On the hand, the reflex is found on the middle of the fleshy muscle at the base of the thumb joint. As both areas are slightly raised, they can be worked from many directions; you can even use your knuckle.

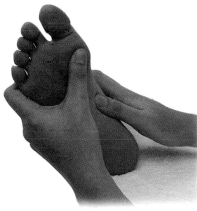

URETERS REFLEX

URETERS REFLEX

Work up the inner edge from zones 1 and into zone 2 to just above the waistline; this pathway follows the line of the ureter reflexes to the kidney point. Work the point several times.

KIDNEY REFLEX

This lays on the sole/palm. In the foot, it is in the central indentation dividing the ball of the foot from the arch, just above the waistline in zones 2 to 3. On the hands, the reflex is at the lowest point of the web, below the adrenal gland reflex. Work the area thoroughly, at least three to six times, but do not apply much pressure, as it is often tender.

WORK AREA
THOROUGHLY

KIDNEY REFLEX

The Reproductive System

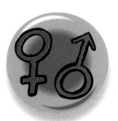

ABOVE *Reflexes for the sexual organs are the same for both sexes.*

THE REPRODUCTIVE SYSTEM *comprises both primary sexual organs (which produce the sex cells containing genetic information) and secondary sexual organs. In females, the primary organs are the two ovaries, and the accessory organs include the two fallopian tubes, the uterus, and the milk-producing mammary glands. In males, the primary organs are the testes; the prostate gland is an accessory glandular organ, as are the vas deferens.*

The female ovaries produce the female sex cells (the eggs) and the hormones progesterone and estrogen, which control the menstrual cycle. The fallopian tubes are the ducts that conduct the eggs to the womb, where fertilization takes place at the ovarian end of the duct. The womb, a hollow organ with a thick lining, is where the fetus develops, and the placenta forms to enable the growing organism to obtain nourishment from the mother. In males, the testes produce

the male sex cells (sperm) and the hormone testosterone, which controls male sexual and physical characteristics; the prostate gland secretes the fluid semen, which contains the sperm cells, while the vas deferens are ducts down which the sperm travel to the urethra.

The reflexes to the reproductive areas are on the top (dorsal) surfaces of the foot and hand, and around the ankle and wrist. The reflexes for the vas deferens in males are in the same location as the reflexes for the

fallopian tubes in females. Similarly, the reflexes for the female ovaries are in the same place as the reflexes for the male testes. Reflexes for the prostate and the uterus are also found in the same place. Treatment helps to balance any hormonal disturbance that is causing menstrual disorders and helps alleviate any pelvic inflammatory problems. In both sexes, it helps to reduce inflammation in the reproductive tract, improving the rich nerve and blood supply to stimulate normal functioning.

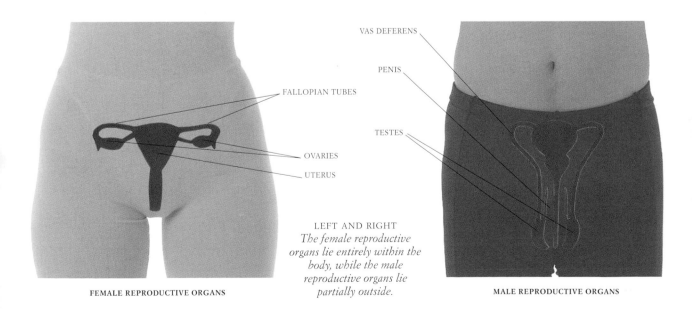

FALLOPIAN TUBES

OVARIES

UTERUS

VAS DEFERENS

PENIS

TESTES

LEFT AND RIGHT
The female reproductive organs lie entirely within the body, while the male reproductive organs lie partially outside.

FEMALE REPRODUCTIVE ORGANS

MALE REPRODUCTIVE ORGANS

REPRODUCTIVE REFLEXES

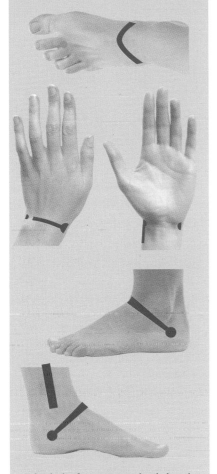

Individual reflex points are detailed on the charts in Appendix One (pp.130–35).

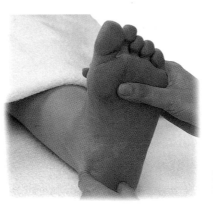

**UTERUS/PROSTATE REFLEXES
MEDIAL SIDE**

REPRODUCTIVE REFLEXES

These are in the depressions on each side of the ankle or wrist – the uterus/prostate on the inner edge, the ovaries/testes on the outer edge. These areas can be worked using either the thumbs or index fingers in all directions. To apply extra stimulation to the two reflex points simultaneously, use the thumb on the outside reflex point and middle finger on the inner reflex, and rotate the person's foot or hand both ways.

BREAST REFLEX

In females, this is in a wide area in zones 2/3 on the top surface of the foot and the back of the hand.

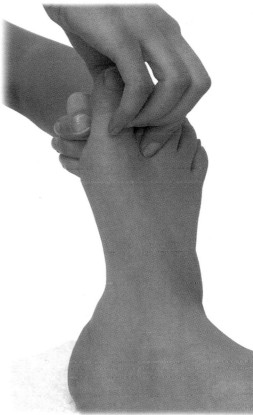

BREAST REFLEX

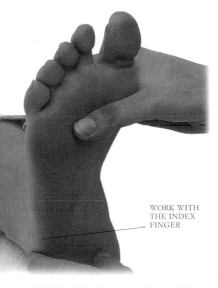

WORK WITH THE INDEX FINGER

OVARIES/TESTES REFLEX: LATERAL SIDE

FALLOPIAN TUBES/VAS DEFERENS

These reflexes form a line across the upper (dorsal) surfaces of the ankle and wrist, linking the above reflexes together. To work these and relax the entire area, overclasp the hands on this line and the reflex for the groin lymphatics just above them (see p. 61). Using the web of one hand in a firm, unmoving pressure, again rotate the foot or hand in an inward direction. You can also work this line with both thumbs, working up from the ankles/wrist to meet on the top of the foot or hand. (Be careful not to pinch the skin.)

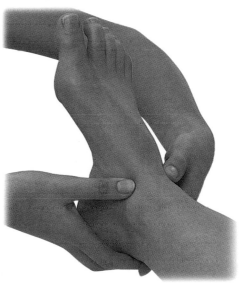

FALLOPIAN/VAS DEFERENS REFLEXES

The Musculoskeletal and Nervous Systems

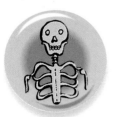

ABOVE *Reflexology aids coordinated movement and relieves sore muscles.*

THE MUSCULOSKELETAL AND NERVOUS SYSTEMS *include the complex network of bones, joints and connective tissues, muscles, and nerves that allow us to move. The musculoskeletal system encompasses not only the bones themselves, but also the muscles that contract to move them and the structures binding the two together. The neurological system comprises the brain, the spinal cord, the nerves running from these organs, major nerve plexuses (nerve clumps), and the peripheral nerves.*

The bones provide a framework for the human body. They are linked together by ligaments. Muscles are attached to the bones by tendons.

In the nervous system, the brain is the coordination and command center (*see p. 46*) From the hindbrain, nerve pathways descend to the muscles and organs. The spinal cord, a continuation of the brain stem, handles reflex reactions.

The reflexes to the musculoskeletal and nervous areas lie along all four edges of the foot and hand. Generally speaking, the spine is represented by the inner (medial) and the arms and legs by the outer (lateral) edges. The reflexes to muscles of the trunk traverse the top (dorsal) surface, while on the lower surface they lie in front of the waistline.

Treatment relieves muscle spasm and aids coordinated movement by

RIGHT *This illustration shows the main muscle areas, but there are over 650 muscles in the human body.*

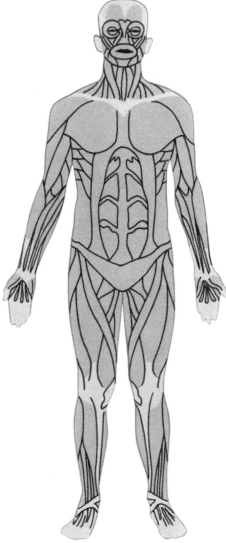

calming the electrical signals originating in the brain that travel down the spinal cord, encouraging relaxation of muscles, ligaments, and tendons. As the brain and spinal cord conveys information to the whole body, treatment stimulates not only these structures, but also has a knock-on effect on the peripheral and autonomic nervous systems interrelating with all the sensory organs, and all the skin and muscles of the body, so it is useful as a general first-aid treatment. Working the foot or hand reflex positions for the cervical nerves can aid most hand and arm problems, while working the reflexes for the lumbar and sacral nerves can aid most leg problems; this is because of the spinal innervation to the upper and lower limbs. For the back, reflexology treatment brings about quick relief and in many cases strengthens the back and vulnerable muscles. (*see pp. 76–77 for back-strengthening exercises*).

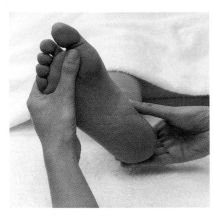

SPINAL REFLEXES

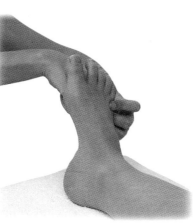

SHOULDER REFLEXES

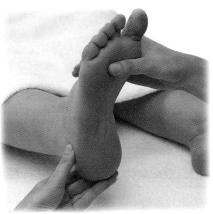

HIP/LEG REFLEXES

SPINAL REFLEXES

These extend from the cervical spine to the tailbone, all the way down the inner edge of the foot and hand, from the base of the nail bed down to the base of the foot and heel.

LIMB REFLEXES

The limb reflexes are on the outer edge of the foot and hand.
(i) The shoulder reflexes run from the fourth and fifth digits to the diaphragm line.
(ii) The arms are between the diaphragm line and the waist reflex.
(iii) The elbow/knee reflex point is on the waistline (on the foot, the bony bulge just behind the midfoot).

HIP REFLEXES

From the waistline to the base of the heel and hand are found the hip and leg-related areas. The reflexes for the muscles of the pelvis and buttocks are found all around the heel and the two padded areas on the base of the hand.

SCIATIC NERVE

On the feet, from the heel base and up the lateral side of the leg. On the hand, where the wrist meets the hand's heel.

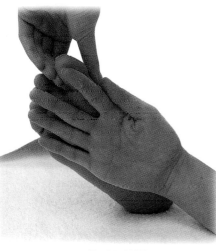

SPINE REFLEX

SHOULDER/ARM REFLEX

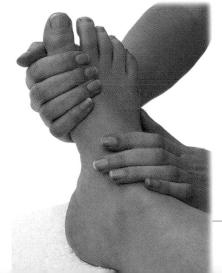

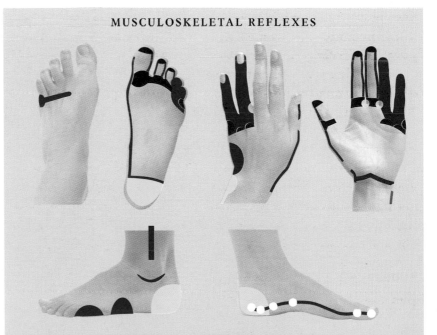

MUSCULOSKELETAL REFLEXES

Individual reflex points are detailed on the charts in Appendix One (pp.130–35).

The Circulatory and Immune Systems

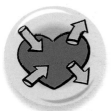

ABOVE *The circulatory system pumps blood around the body.*

THE BLOOD CIRCULATORY SYSTEM *includes the heart itself and the blood circulation network. The immune system comprises the lymph nodes and lymph circulation network, the spleen, and the thymus.*

In the circulatory system, the heart is a powerful pump, rhythmically contracting in response to nerve impulses originating within the heart itself. The system of blood vessels comprises arteries (carrying blood from the heart), a network of small capillaries, and veins (returning blood to the heart). In the immune system, the thymus gland is the primary organ, producing immune cells called lymphocytes (white blood cells), while the spleen is a secondary organ that processes incoming blood, filters out damaged cells, and destroys foreign substances; it also helps produce antibodies (which fight invading organisms).

NOTE

Reflexology treatment improves the function of the many lymphatic valves, improves filtration and absorption of waste products, and can only stimulate and aid immunity.

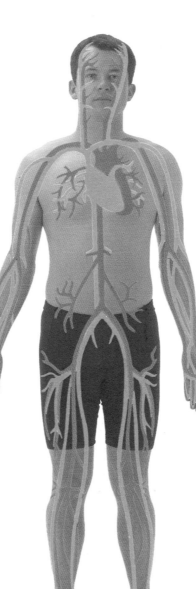

The reflexes for the blood circulation system are found on the lower surfaces at the front of the foot and hand. Those for the immune system are located on the top (dorsal) surfaces. Treatment improves the blood circulation generally by providing nervous stimulation and increases lymph drainage, therefore helping to transport both vital nutrients and hormones to tissues as well as getting rid of waste products. Extra stimulation of the spleen and thymus areas is essential in infective conditions, as spleen stimulation encourages the destruction of invading microbes, while thymus enhancement activates cells that respond to entry of foreign substances. The thymus is largest in infancy, declining in size as maturity is reached.

LEFT *The circulatory system is composed of the heart, blood vessels, and the blood. Fresh oxygenated blood is conducted away from the heart, carrying oxygen and nutrients to organs and tissues in the body. The deoxygenated blood then returns to the heart via the veins in order to be reoxygenated in the lungs.*

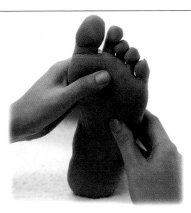

SPLEEN REFLEX

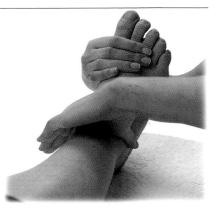

LOWER LYMPHATICS/GROIN REFLEX

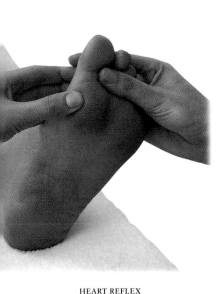

HEART REFLEX

HEART REFLEX

On the left foot, this reflex is on the ball of the foot, stretching over zones 1 and 2; on the right foot, however, it is only in zone 1. Also, on the left hand it is only in zone 2. Working from this area across to the little toe or finger aids the whole circulatory system, as both lungs and heart are then contacted.

THYMUS REFLEX

SPLEEN REFLEX

The spleen reflex is on the left foot only, its base in contact with the tail of the pancreas reflex, in zones 4 to 5.

UPPER LYMPHATICS

The reflexes to the upper (neck and shoulder) lymphatics are found in the webs between the bases of the fingers and toes. Work these by making a fist of your supporting hand. Now place the thumb of the working hand loosely in between the thumb and forefinger of the support hand, giving a pincer action. Work with the fingers across the webs of the toes or fingers, starting from the great toe or thumb and moving toward the little toe/finger.

UPPER LYMPHATICS REFLEX

LOWER LYMPHATICS

The reflexes to the lower lymphatics form a line across the dorsal surface of the foot/hand, between the ankle/wrist bones, on the line of the vas deferens/ fallopian tubes (see p. 57). Work these by overclasping the hands on this line and, using the web of one hand in a firm, unmoving pressure, rotate the foot or hand in an inward direction.

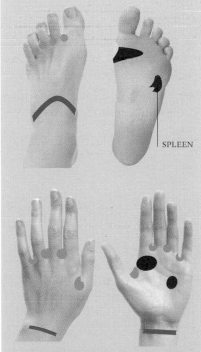

CIRCULATORY REFLEXES

SPLEEN

Individual reflex points are detailed on the charts in Appendix One (pp.130–35).

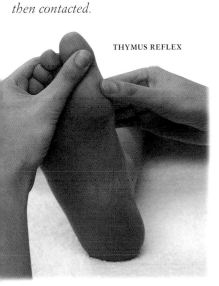

THYMUS REFLEX

This is found on the inner edge, just above the heart reflex.

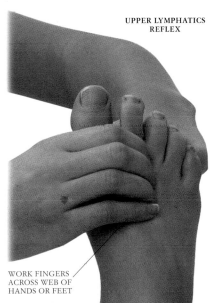

WORK FINGERS ACROSS WEB OF HANDS OR FEET

Auricular Therapy

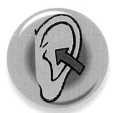

ABOVE *Self ear massage is easy and very beneficial.*

AURICULAR OR EAR MASSAGE *on oneself is simple, and there are no contraindications to this treatment; it can be carried out very easily and without discomfort, even on the very elderly, tiny babies, and animals. Ear therapy developed from early Chinese practice, which held that the shape of the ear reflected a person's health.*

According to the Chinese, the shape of the ear lobe is linked to a person's make-up. When the lobe is long and broad, it is indicative of good health and strong kidneys. If, conversely, the lobe is short and thin, this indicates that the person has a weak constitution. Modern auricular therapy developed from early Chinese diagnostic techniques. At one time there were over 230 different acupoints in the ear being used for treatment. Practitioners now use a combination of Dr. Nogier's theory (*see pp. 16–17*) and T.C.M. Over a period, the therapy has received increasing international recognition and is now widely practiced in many countries. In more recent years it has become more precise.

In 1982, the World Health Organization (W.H.O.), along with the Chinese Acupuncture and Moxibustion Association, formulated a standard set of points known as I.S.A.P. There are 90 points listed in the I.S.A.P. (*see Appendix One, pp. 130–135*).

Of the nerves that supply the ear, an important one is the vagus nerve (known as the wanderer, because of its far-reaching effects in the body),

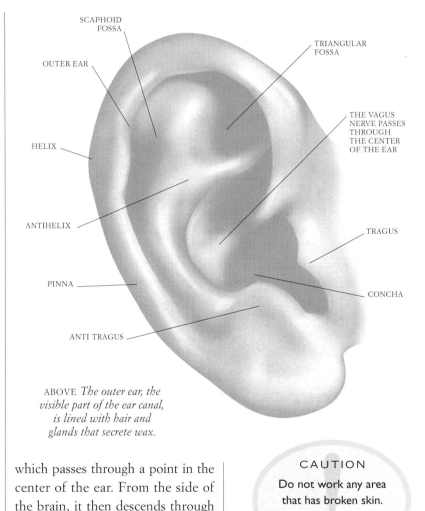

SCAPHOID FOSSA

OUTER EAR

HELIX

ANTIHELIX

PINNA

ANTI TRAGUS

TRIANGULAR FOSSA

THE VAGUS NERVE PASSES THROUGH THE CENTER OF THE EAR

TRAGUS

CONCHA

ABOVE *The outer ear, the visible part of the ear canal, is lined with hair and glands that secrete wax.*

which passes through a point in the center of the ear. From the side of the brain, it then descends through the neck and thorax, with branches to the ear, tongue, pharynx, larynx, and gullet, reaching down to the abdominal region. Nearly all nerves send branches to the triangular fossa. Also, many of the Chinese

CAUTION
Do not work any area that has broken skin.

meridians pass around or enter the ear. This is probably why auricular therapy is so successful.

WARM UP

Rub your palms together until they are warm, then massage both the front and back ear surfaces between them. Using your thumb and finger, work in little circles or press together on both the back and the front surface. Pressure should only be as much as the person can bear comfortably. Use the index finger in all the hollows, as this is the most sensitive of all the fingers.

These procedures should be repeated several times, until the ear is quite hot. This increased stimulation is extremely effective for relieving pain in any part of the body.

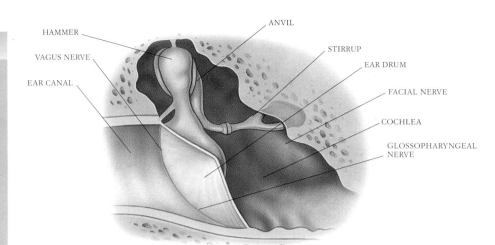

ABOVE *An awareness of the workings of the inner ear helps you to understand the effects of auricular therapy.*

ANATOMY AND PHYSIOLOGY OF THE EAR

In shape the ears resemble the kidneys, and in T.C.M. the two are considered to be closely linked. Also, if we look at the brain and the cerebrum, with its deep convolutions, and its representative areas in the sensory and motor cortex, we see a similar arrangement of body areas depicted on the auricle.

Studying the basic anatomy of the ear enables you to be aware of the physiological effect of auricular therapy.

The main areas are as follows:
• The auricle or pinna is the part on the outside of the head.
• The helix is the rim or roll of cartilage.
• The antihelix is the inner curvature.
• The long, narrow, curved furrow between the helix and the antihelix is called the scapha (or scaphoid fossa).
• The triangular-shaped hollow on the upper ear is called the triangular fossa (fossa means "trench-like").
• The central hollow is called the concha (concha means "shell-like").

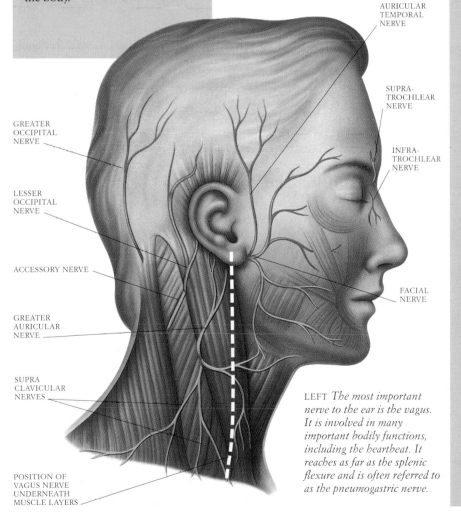

LEFT *The most important nerve to the ear is the vagus. It is involved in many important bodily functions, including the heartbeat. It reaches as far as the splenic flexure and is often referred to as the pneumogastric nerve.*

Ear Treatment Sequence

A FULL EAR MASSAGE *may incorporate a number of specific points, and may be varied according to particular health problems. A good general order of working the ear areas, including the most important points, is as follows:*

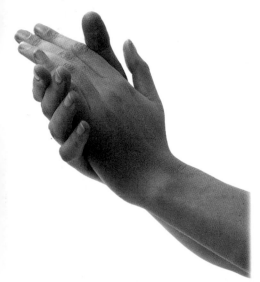

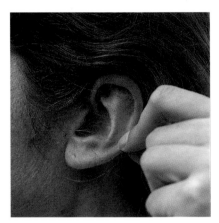

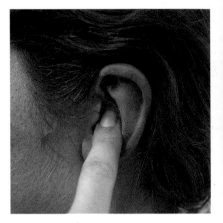

STEP 1 *Before beginning the treatment, make sure to warm up your hands.*

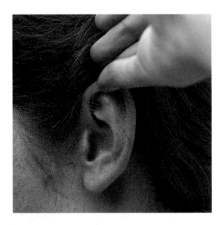

STEP 2 *Squeeze the very top of your ear (fold the flap over to find the reflex point at the top, or apex, of the ear). This treatment is ideal for any inflammatory condition, or any fever, as it has a soothing and analgesic effect on the body.*

STEP 3 *Press and palpate down the six points shown on the outer rim. These are good for all upper respiratory tract infections, inflammation of the tonsils or pharynx, and fevers.*

Just above the first of these are two T.C.M. points: the first (Liver Yang) is good for hypertension, headaches, or dizziness. Slightly above it is a point used for allergic disorders (called "Wind Stream" in T.C.M.); it is also used to treat skin disorders, such as itching, eczema, urticaria (patches of red skin), allergic rhinitis (nasal inflammation), and rheumatoid arthritis.

STEP 4 *Put your finger into a point in the center of the ear (sometimes called "zero point"). This is where the vagus nerve (see p. 63) passes through the ear, and it can be used as a stimulating or sedative point for the parasympathetic nervous system. Refer to Divisions of the Nervous System, (see p. 21). Stimulation here slows the heart down, and helps with any abdominal disorders or pain. This point is also used for neurosis, and for hiccups.*

TIP

Keep your nails clipped to avoid hurting the patient when applying pressure during an ear massage.

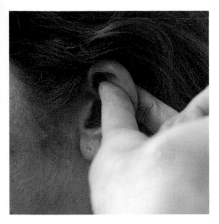

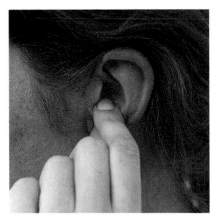

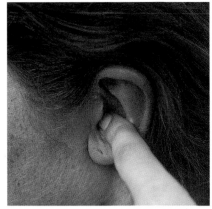

STEP 5 *Work in the upper hollow (triangular fossa). This is a vital area for hypertension as it lowers the blood pressure. It also used for asthma, as it has an antiallergic and antirheumatic action.*

In the same depression is a point ("Ear Shenmen" in T.C.M.) that is used for relieving pain. Put your index finger in the ear and your thumb behind the ear. Press, and pull slightly toward the back of your head. Working all around it will also aid lower back disorders.

STEP 7 *Repeat this method on the second area of projecting cartilage just above the lobe (antitragus). One point here is used for inflammatory problems; it is also useful as an asthma-relieving point. Just behind it is a point relating to the brain stem; it can have either a stimulatory or an inhibitory effect on the cerebral cortex in the forebrain. It is used for any diseases of the nervous, digestive, endocrine, or genitourinary systems, hemorrhage and Menière's syndrome. On the back of this projection is a point that has a powerful analgesic action on the nervous system. This point can be used for any circulatory or functional disorder of the autonomic nervous system.*

STEP 9 *This point at the bottom of the frontal cartilage projection has marvellous anti-inflammatory and antiallergic properties, and is also suitable for rheumatic disorders. This widely used point also regulates both hypertension and hypotension.*

STEP 10 *The point in the crease at the bottom of the concha is used for all menstrual and urogenital problems, diabetes, obesity, and it also has anti-inflammatory properties. It is known as the endocrine or hormone point.*

HOLD BETWEEN THUMB AND INDEX FINGER, MANIPULATING THE WHOLE AREA

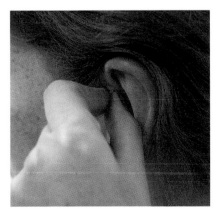

STEP 6 *A point on the projecting cartilage at the front of the ear (tragus) is good for inflammatory disorders, fever, and to relieve pain. Place your thumb behind the protuberance with your index finger on top, and apply pressure.*

STEP 8 *Use your index finger to work in the bowl-shaped cavity (the concha). The first point here (in the angle) relates to inflammation of the prostate and the urethra (see pp. 54–55). It is also ideal to treat any other infections of the urinary tract. The second point, in the center of the upper concha, is for any abdominal pain, or for circulatory disorders.*

ENDOCRINE OR HORMONE POINT

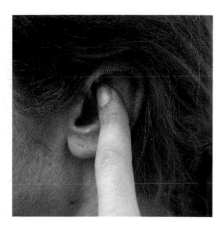

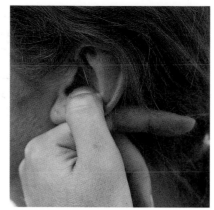

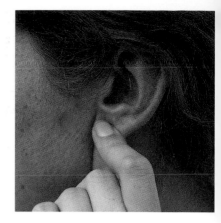

STEP 11 *There are two useful points on the antihelix:*
(i) The body of the antihelix corresponds to the spine, it is the first point to work for any problems of the hip and all sciatic areas.
(ii) Just under the rim is a point specific to the sympathetic nervous system. Applying pressure on this point helps to alleviate any abdominal pain or cramps. However, it should not be used in acute swelling and pain, as it may mask the symptoms and prevent the practitioner from making the correct diagnosis and treatment. This point will also help in any coronary heart disease, spasm, or constriction of arteries or veins. It also inhibits glandular secretion, so it can be used for those suffering from excessive sweating and weeping dermatitis.

STEP 12 *In the indentation above the lobe behind the endocrine point is a point where three major nerves pass through the ear, including the vagus nerve (the vagus nerve is a vagovagal reflex that conveys sensory and motor nerves, see p. 63), and facial nerves, and the nerve supplying the tongue and pharynx. This point (known in T.C.M. as "Triple Burner" or "Sanjiao" point) will aid any problem or pain in the facial area, including paralysis, jaw/cheek nerve pain, and toothache.*

STEP 13 *The anterior lobe of the ear corresponds to the head and facial areas; a point here also acts as an anesthetic point for tooth extraction.*

POINT FOR CENTER OF EAR, ALSO KNOWN AS THE STIMULATING POINT FOR THE VAGUS NERVE

ZERO OR CENTER POINT

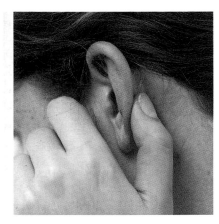

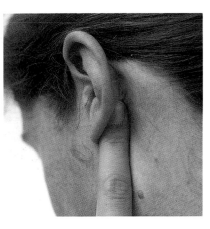

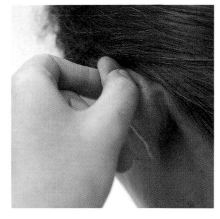

STEP 14 *The back (dorsal surface) of the ear also contains ten useful reflex points:*
(i) Just stroking the center back of the ear achieves a beneficial effect on many parts of the body, as the root of the vagus nerve passes through at this point.

(iii) At the bottom of the ear is a point used for noises in the ear, or tinnitus (which is known in T.C.M. as "Yang Wei").
(iv) The point on the lower ear root is ideal to aid low blood pressure (hypotension).

(v) This point in the groove balances blood pressure.
(vi) The heart point is for insomnia, nightmares, and palpitations (see p. 135).
(vii) The lung point is useful for all bronchial problems (see p. 135).
(viii) The spleen point (see p. 135) is for indigestion and stomach pain; it also stimulates the appetite and is an ideal point for improving anorexia.
(ix) The liver point (see p. 135) is for any pain in the side areas of the abdomen.
(x) The kidney point (see p. 135) is used to correct any tendency toward neurosis, dizziness, or headaches.

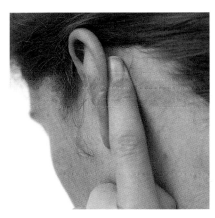

THE DORSAL SURFACE OF THE EAR HAS TEN USEFUL REFLEX POINTS

(ii) Further toward the top of the ear is a reflex point for the spinal cord; it is used for paralysis of the face or arm. As this is caused by a malfunction in the opposite hemisphere of the brain, work the ear point on the opposite side from the paralysis.

Treatment of the Face and Head

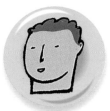

ABOVE *Acupressure is extremely beneficial for facial areas.*

ACUPRESSURE CAN BE USED *on all areas of the face, with very beneficial results. Massage and palpation on specific points of the head are particularly stimulating to the brain, eyes, ears, and face. It is a wonderful and easy way of relieving the many physical symptoms of stress – tension headaches can disappear, mood is enhanced and balanced, concentration is aided, and impaired sleep patterns generally improve. It also enhances the skin circulation and the complexion, brightens the eyes, and can sharpen vision. Most of the body's internal organs can be stimulated.*

FACIAL ACUPRESSURE

Facial massage is so rejuvenating because it covers many important pressure points. We often use acupressure unknowingly to relieve tension, as you can see in the following examples:

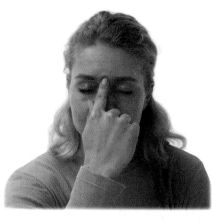

MIDDLE OF EYEBROWS POINT
How often, when we are concentrating, do we put our index finger in the middle of the eyebrows? The point we press by this action is used for calming the mind.

INNER CORNERS OF EYES
We often press the inner corners of the eyes when they are tired. The ophthalmic nerve, running to the eyeball, eyelid, tear ducts, sinuses, and forehead, passes under this point (see p. 71).

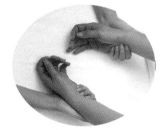

SHENMEN POINT
When a person is hysterical, how often do we instinctively grab them by their wrists? This point is known as a calming point, in T.C.M. called "Shenmen" ("Spirit's Door").

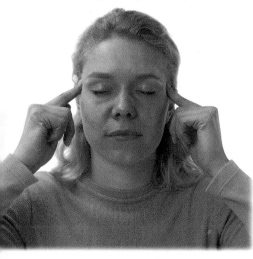

TEMPLES POINT
Many people automatically press the sides of their temples when they have a headache or migraine. This pressure will relieve nerve congestion and irritation in the temporal nerve, which runs to the jaw and temples.

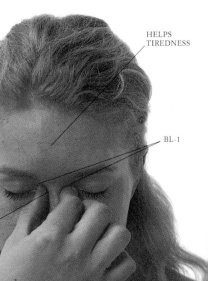

HELPS TIREDNESS

BL-1

PRESS CORNERS OF EYES

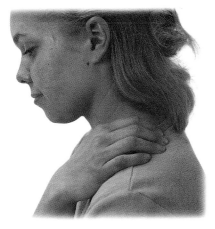

SHOULDER POINT
Often, if our shoulders are stiff or tense, we press or massage our shoulder muscle. We are working a point that is considered perfect for all shoulder and neck problems.

BELOW *The points on the face and head are known as Ah Shi points in T.C.M (see pp. 136–40).*

AH SHI POINTS

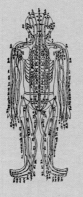

Points on the face and head include those known in T.C.M. as "Ah Shi" (the Chinese for "oh, yes") points, which are sore spots revealed by palpation or pressure. The theory behind their use was first developed by Sun Si Miao during the Tang dynasty (C.E. 581–682), who stated that at these points the meridians came particularly close and effectively merged, so that many meridians could be affected by using them. They are now known to coincide generally with musculoskeletal "trigger points," which are activated by referred nerve activity (*see p. 82*).

ABOVE *The theory of acupressure was first developed by the Chinese in the sixth century.*

FACIAL POINTS AND MERIDIANS

The points on the face are beneficial because they incorporate points on all six Yang meridians (*see p. 12*). The three Yang meridians of the hands ascend to the face, while the three Yang meridians of the feet descend from the face. Two other vital meridians, the Conception Vessel and the Governor Vessel, circle the midline of the body in opposite directions to terminate on the face below and above the mouth, respectively (*see p. 140*).

So the face has many terminating and originating points connecting to the different organ systems. At such points, the energy is believed to be particularly easy to contact. Many of these points are also located over or near major nerves in the area (*see p. 63*). Stimulating these points daily is extremely advantageous, as they not only help tone the internal organs, but also calm the mind. They also improve the tone of the facial muscles generally.

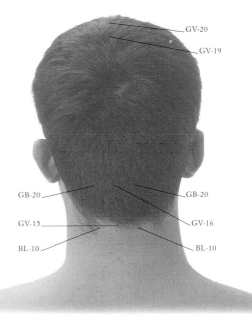

EX-2
GB-14
EX-3
BL-2
TB-23
EX-5
GB-1
SI-19
ST-1
EX-6
ST-2
BL-1
LI-20
CV-24

GB-14
EX-3
BL-2
TB-23
EX-5
GB-1
SI-19
ST-1
EX-6
ST-2
BL-1
LI-20
GV-26

GV-20
GV-19

GB-20
GV-15
BL-10

GB-20
GV-16
BL-10

Pressure Points to Use on the Face and Head

AS A DAILY HEALTH EXERCISE, *the following pressure points can be pressed and palpated (squeezed) for at least 30 seconds. However, if there is any severe discomfort with a particular point, it is best to discontinue the pressure immediately.*

POINTS AROUND THE EYE AREA

There are several extremely beneficial points around the eye area that can help alleviate headaches, dizziness, trigeminal neuralgia, insomnia, or just aid relaxation of tired eyes.

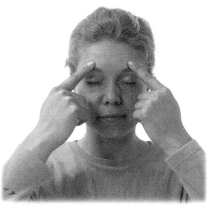

GB-14 REFLEX

GB-14
One finger-width above the midline of each eyebrow is a point on the Gallbladder meridian (the 14th point, abbreviated to GB-14). It is useful for all types of headache, as well as jaw and cheek pain (trigeminal neuralgia).

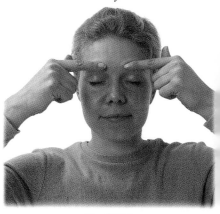

BL-2 REFLEX

BL-2
On the inner edge of each eyebrow is a point on the Bladder meridian (BL-2). This is a point for treating "floaters" in the eyes, glaucoma, headaches, and trigeminal neuralgia.

PRESS BETWEEN THE EYEBROWS

THIS IS A GOOD POINT FOR RELIEVING HEADACHES

THE SEVENTH CRANIAL NERVE SERVES THIS AREA

YINGTANG POINT
On the midline of the face between both of the eyebrows is a point that is also useful for all headaches, insomnia, dizziness, and nasal problems.

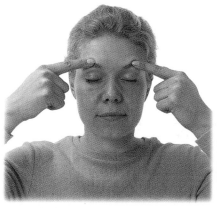

YUYAO POINT

YUYAO POINT
On the middle of each eyebrow (immediately below point GB-14) is a point that is good for conjunctivitis, or for just relaxing the eyes.

TEMPLE POINT

One finger-width behind the outside edge of each eyebrow (in the depression) is a point that can be used for all facial problems, plus headaches, migraines, trigeminal neuralgia, and toothache. The facial nerve serves this point.

PLACE FINGERS ON OUTSIDE EDGE OF EYEBROW

USED TO RELIEVE TOOTHACHE

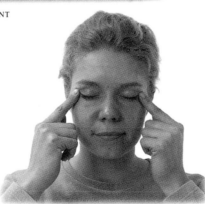

TEMPLE POINT

BL-1

In the depression just above the inner corner of the eye is the first point on the Bladder meridian (BL-1). This point can be used for treating many eye disorders, such as conjunctivitis, near-sightedness (myopia), glaucoma, and inflammation of the retina (the reflective layer at the back of the eye). It is popularly known as "eye brightness."

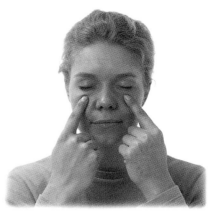

ST-1 REFLEX

ST-1

On the bone just below the eye, in line with pupil, is the first point on the Stomach meridian (ST-1). It is an ideal point for all eye problems, such as tired eyes, redness, or any degeneration of vision, such as near-sightedness. This particular point is very near to the surface and is rich in blood vessels, so light tapping is all that is needed.

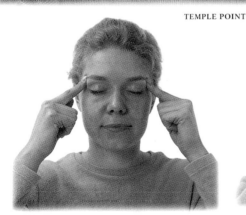

TB-23 REFLEX

TB-23

On the outside edge side of each eyebrow is found the last point on the Triple Burner meridian (TB-23). It is useful for headaches, facial problems, and conjunctivitis.

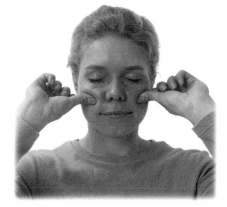

GB-1 REFLEX

GB-1

On the outer corner of the eye lies the first point on the Gallbladder meridian (GB-1). This point is also suitable for all eye disorders, as BL-1 above, and migraines.

ST-2 REFLEX

ST-2

Immediately below point ST-1 (see above) is the second point on the Stomach meridian (ST-2). It is a good point for alleviating all eye disorders, and for any facial spasms or trigeminal neuralgia. It greatly eases the discomfort of conjunctivitis.

POINTS AROUND THE NOSE AND MOUTH

There are many useful points around the nose and mouth area, which may be used daily to relieve irritating or uncomfortable ailments. Problems that can be helped by stimulating these points include constipation, tinnitus, sinusitis, and depression.

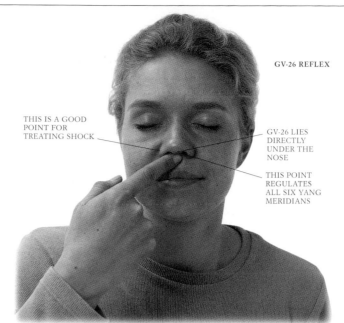

GV-26 REFLEX

THIS IS A GOOD POINT FOR TREATING SHOCK

GV-26 LIES DIRECTLY UNDER THE NOSE

THIS POINT REGULATES ALL SIX YANG MERIDIANS

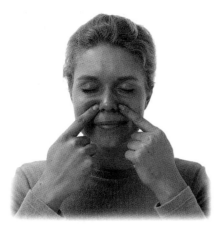

LI-20 REFLEX

LI-20

This point, which lies in the crease as you smile as near to the nose as possible, is the last point on the Large Intestine meridian (LI-20). It is a good point for all nasal problems, sinusitis, allergic rhinitis, and loss of the sense of smell. It is also an ideal point to stem a bleeding nose (while leaning forward). Finally, it can relieve trigeminal neuralgia.

SI-19

This point lies in the depression formed next to the ear when you open your mouth. It is the last point on the Small Intestine meridian (SI-19). It is frequently used for all ear disorders, including ringing in the ears (tinnitus), weeping inflammation, deafness, and toothaches.

GV-26

This point lies in the midline directly under the nose and is the last point on the Governor Vessel channel (GV-26), which in T.C.M. is considered to regulate the energy of all six Yang meridians. It is excellent for treating fainting and unconsciousness, shock, and is a major point for aiding mental disorders and epilepsy. It is used as an empirical point for acute lower back problems, where the cause lies in the backbones themselves. Applying pressure on this point (push up on the midline of the depression) will aid movement when standing and arching the back.

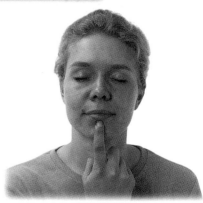

CV-24 REFLEX

CV-24

This point lies on the middle of the lower lip, and is the last point on the Conception Vessel channel. It is ideal for constipation and all reproductive imbalances. This point can also be used for dry mouth (xerostomia), and trigeminal neuralgia. It also regulates all the yin channels.

SI-19 REFLEX

NOTE

Dr. Joe Shelby-Riley advocated the use of the CV-24 point for constipation, stating, "Press with fingertips into the chin for 7 or 8 minutes."

POINTS ON THE BACK OF THE HEAD AND NECK

On the back of the head and neck are several points that can aid minor problems. These sites aid in clarifying the mind and increasing the vitality, so they are ideal to use when a person is depressed.

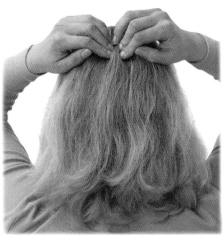

GV-19 REFLEX

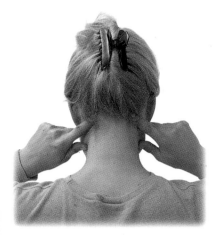

GB-20 REFLEX

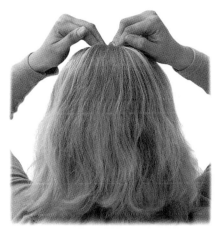

GV-20

On the highest point of the head is a point on the Governor Vessel that is called "Baihui" in T.C.M., meaning "Hundred Meetings." This is because the Yang meridians meet at this point. It is ideal for headaches including migraines, dizziness, lightheadedness, or vertigo. It is also very calming, so is useful for mental tension and anxiety.

GV-19

Two finger-widths below GV-20 is another point on the same channel that is useful for headaches, cerebral congestion, and vertigo. It is also a good calming point for anxiety. Use both the index and middle fingers of both hands together to apply pressure on each of the above points, and move the scalp gently around in a circular movement several times.

GV-16

In the center of the nape of the neck, just above the hair line, is a third point on the Governor Vessel. It is used for headaches, to clear the mind and clarify the thoughts, and is helpful in mental disorders. Rotate on this point for a few minutes.

GB-20

This point is known in T.C.M. as the "Fengchi" or "Wind" point. It is used to release Qi that is trapped in the head to return it back down to the lower body. It helps congestive conditions in the head and neck, including pains or any stiffness in the neck, eye disorders, head colds, nasal inflammation, ringing in the ears, and hypertension.

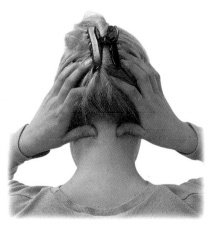

BL-10 REFLEX

BL-10

Just below GB-20 and slightly nearer to the midline on each side of the head is a point on the Bladder meridian (BL-10). This is a vital point for headaches, stiff necks, and it can help a sore throat. It is also good for lower back problems.

GV-16 REFLEX

ROTATE FINGER ON GV-16

GOOD FOR MENTAL DISORDERS

Exercises for the Foot, Hand, and Back

A NUMBER OF EXERCISES *can be followed on a daily basis to give a general toning stimulation to the hand and foot reflex areas; this provides an easy and quick routine for health maintenance. There are also exercises that can be followed to strengthen the spine, stimulate the spinal nerves, and relieve back pain.*

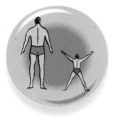

ABOVE *Daily exercise will help to keep the body in a supple and healthy condition.*

FOOT AND HAND EXERCISES

Try to do at least some of these easy exercises daily to keep your hands and feet in a healthy condition.

EXERCISE 1 *Shake the hands or feet, and rotate the ankles or wrists both ways.*

EXERCISE 2 *Wriggle and stretch your toes, fanning and separating them as much as possible. Do the same with your fingers, clenching your fists then fanning your fingers out, extending them as much as possible. This exercise aids the head and neck area, and also the lower back.*

EXERCISE 3 *Extend the great toe as much as possible, point the toe, then bend it upward. Repeat with the thumb, or use a rubber band on the thumb and little finger, stretching it as much as possible. This exercise specifically aids the neck area.*

EXERCISE 4 *For the feet only: turn them inward so the soles face each other, then turn them outward. This exercise is good for the spinal column.*

BELOW *Exercise 4 is ideal for the spinal column.*

EXERCISE 5 *Walk on the heels of the feet. This exercise aids the lower back.*

WALK ON HEELS OF FEET

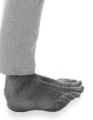

ABOVE *If you suffer from lower back pain, try doing this exercise.*

FIRST TURN FEET INWARD

THEN TURN FEET OUTWARD

PLACE BALL
UNDER FOOT
AND ROLL

PICK UP PENCIL
WITH YOUR TOES

CLASP HANDS
TOGETHER AND
PRESS DOWN
INTO THE WEBS

ABOVE *This simple
exercise helps the neck
and shoulder areas.*

ABOVE *Roll a ball to
stimulate the respiratory
and digestive tracts.*

ABOVE *Try this exercise
if you have tired hands.*

EXERCISE 6 *Walk on the balls of the
feet. This exercise aids the lungs and
is very good for asthmatics.*

EXERCISE 7 *Try to pick up a pencil
with your toes. This exercise aids the
neck and shoulder areas.*

EXERCISE 8 *Place a ball or other
round object under your feet and roll
it the length of the foot; repeat this
two or three times. This stimulates
the respiratory and digestive tracts.*

EXERCISE 9 *For tired hands, clasp
the hands together and press down
into the webs.*

EXERCISE 10 *For tired legs and
feet, assume a comfortable sitting
position, and place a twisted towel
under the arch of the foot. Hold both
ends, pull gently, straightening the
leg and lifting; this is a gentle stretch
for the Achilles tendon.*

EXERCISE 11 *Apply pressure on the
top of your foot by placing one foot
on top of the other. Press the top one
down and pull the bottom one up.
This is very good for the spine and
legs and also aids the lung area.*

EXERCISE 12 *To benefit the hands,
press them together and hold for at
least 60 seconds.*

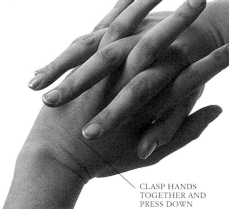

PULL GENTLY

THIS WILL
STRETCH THE
ACHILLES
TENDON

TWISTED
TOWEL

RIGHT *Exercise 10
is beneficial for tired
legs and feet.*

EXERCISES
FOR THE BACK

Do these back-stretching exercises
when you get up in the morning.

BEND KNEES

ARCH BACK
CONCAVELY

EXERCISE 1 *Bending your
knees so that the soles of your
feet are flat on the floor, arch
your back concavely as if you
were trying to push it down
through the floor; repeat this
several times.*

LEFT *Warm up your
back muscles with this
gentle exercise.*

EXERCISE 2 *Raise each leg
separately as near to your chest as
possible, then try it with both knees.*

RAISE BOTH KNEES
TO THE CHEST

LIE FACE DOWN
ON FLOOR

ABOVE AND BELOW
*This exercise will
help strengthen your
back muscles.*

EXERCISE 3 *Raise one foot 6–8in.
from floor, keeping hips in contact
with the floor at all times. Make
sure you do not arch your back.*

SLOW, CONTROLLED
MOVEMENTS

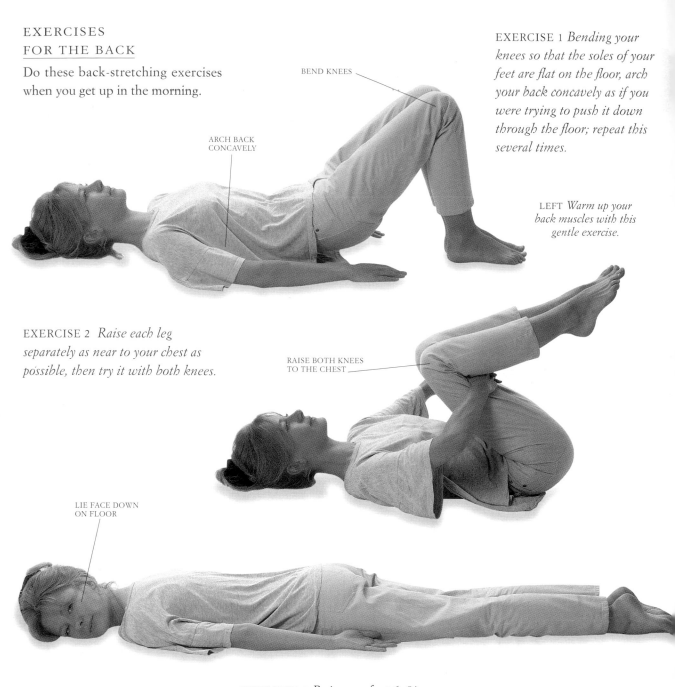

76

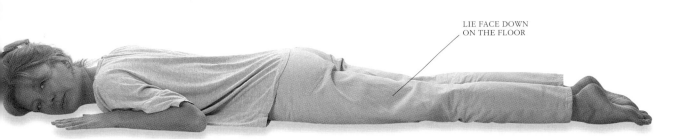

LIE FACE DOWN
ON THE FLOOR

EXERCISE 4 *Keeping your forearms on the floor, gently raise the upper body. This back extension exercise will help strengthen your back.*

ABOVE AND BELOW
This is another excellent exercise for the back muscles.

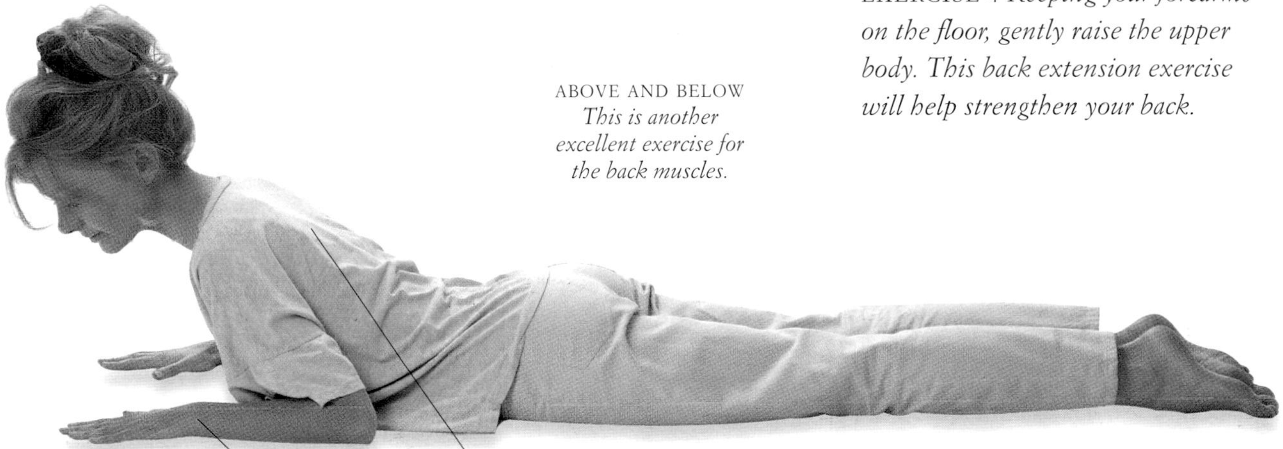

KEEP FOREARMS
AND HANDS ON
THE FLOOR

KEEP HEAD IN LINE
WITH THE SPINE

EXERCISE 5 *Place feet flat on the floor. Pull in your abdominal muscles and then roll your knees down toward the floor. Repeat to the opposite side.*

EXERCISE 6 *Stretch your head gently to the right. You will feel the stretch up the opposite side of the neck. Repeat to the left side. Always move the neck very slowly when you are exercising.*

PULL IN
STOMACH
MUSCLES

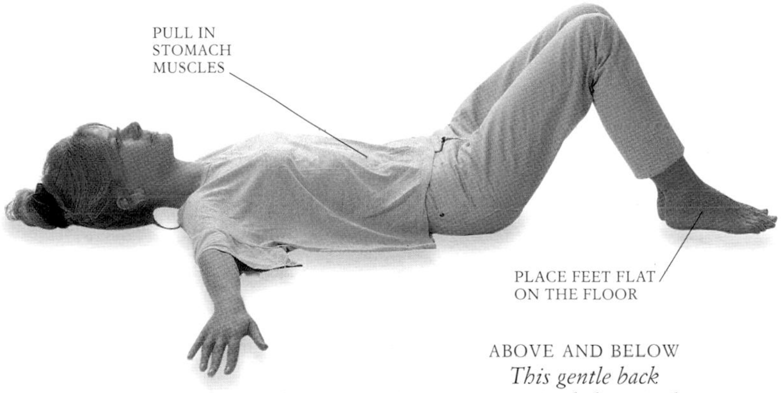

PLACE FEET FLAT
ON THE FLOOR

ABOVE AND BELOW
This gentle back exercise helps spinal flexibility.

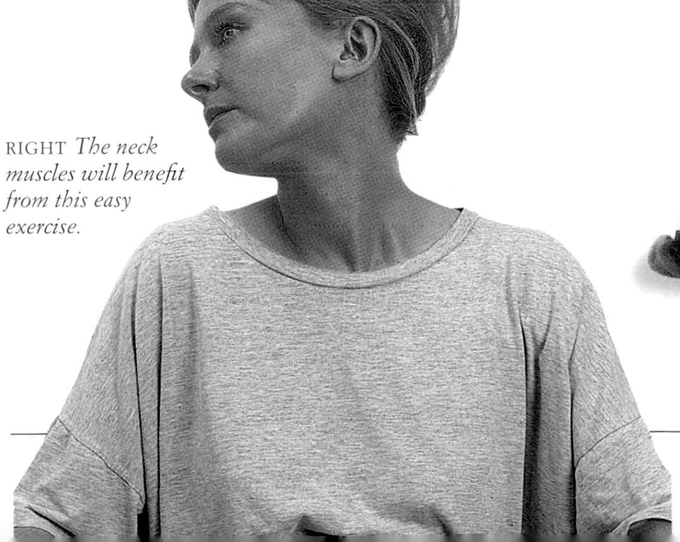

ROLL KNEES OVER
TO ONE SIDE

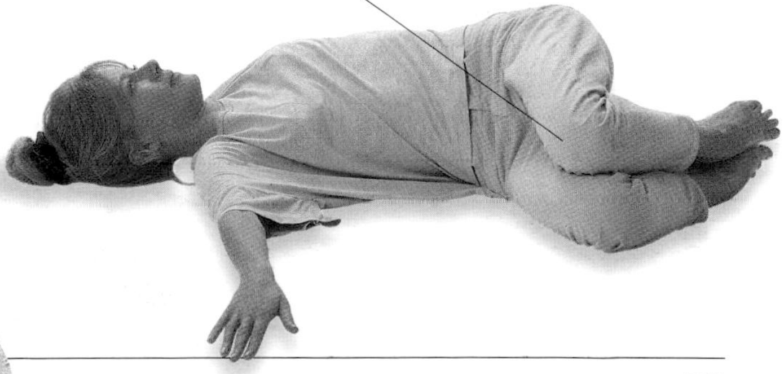

RIGHT *The neck muscles will benefit from this easy exercise.*

Reflexology for Common Problems

THERE ARE A VARIETY *of common conditions for which reflexology will provide specific relief. This section describes the methods of working, as well as any specific indications and body areas to concentrate on for a number of complaints. Along with the foot and hand reflexes, some useful related acupoints on the ear and head are also given here. Specific foods may also alleviate or aggravate the condition, so some useful dietary tips are added where appropriate.*

LEFT *Specific problems may be helped by treatment on the hands.*

Over the years, reflexology has proved highly successful in diagnosing imbalances thus helping with medical problems that are both widespread and commonplace. When assessing how reflexology can help, we need to look at the ways in which disease can affect and enter the body. We do not catch a bad back or headache, constipation or irritable bowel syndrome: they are just a few of the many conditions that may manifest themselves due to our lifestyle, and which reflexology treatment can help.

BELOW *Repetitive strain injury, usually caused by continual use of a computer keyboard, can be helped by reflexology.*

It is imperative to cultivate a healthy mind and body. The old adages "we are what we eat" and "we are what we do" are plain common sense. Worry, stress, and anxiety account for a significant proportion of current health problems because they all weaken our nerve force and lower our vitality. If your mind is positively directed and you establish and maintain good health habits, it will have a wonderful healing influence on your whole body.

According to Chinese philosophy, the emotions play a very important role in the maintenance of health and prevention of illness. T.C.M. contends that the emotions are linked to the five solid (Yin) organs of the body known as the Zang (comprising

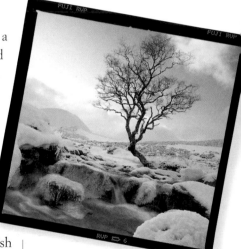

ABOVE *Some common complaints, such as bladder problems, may be aggravated by cold weather.*

the Lungs, Heart, Spleen, Liver, and Kidneys), which are thought to be linked to all the fundamental substances of the body and how they are regulated, stored, and manufactured. If the emotions become unbalanced over a period of time, the physical body will degenerate accordingly.

Laughter and sleep are Nature's medicine. Laughter stimulates certain centers in the brain that control the emotions. A chemical reaction is triggered by an electrical nerve impulse and the brain's natural endorphins, or tranquilizers, are released. Because endorphins have great painkilling qualities, they effectively relieve any feelings of anxiety, but at the same time the blood supply to every organ in the body is improved, generating a feeling of well-being.

Likewise, when a person is tickled, the specialized finer nerve endings that lie just beneath the surface of the skin are excited, with the nerve endings in the palms and soles of the feet being particularly sensitive. The compression of tissue that results brings about an immediate reaction: the pulse usually quickens, blood flow is improved, and whole body appears to respond.

BELOW *Reflexology can help to alleviate sore muscles or rheumatic pain.*

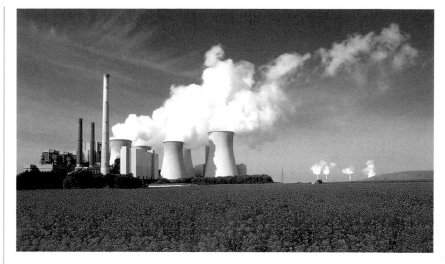

ABOVE *Pollution can cause damaging respiratory problems. However, these often respond well to reflexology treatment.*

If you are deprived of sleep due to anxiety, worry, or ill-health, you function far less efficiently. Sleep is the body's restorative. While we sleep, the parasympathetic nervous system (one of the two divisions of our autonomic nervous system) controls our internal systems, helping to create the conditions needed for rest, sleep, and digestion, and preparing us for the following day.

There are many different categories of disease: viral, bacterial, parasitic, and autoimmune disorders, the latter occurring when the body loses its ability to protect itself because it does not recognize its own antibodies, and this results in inflammation and destruction of tissues. For all of these problems, the practice of reflexology offers an holistic approach, whereby the patient's physical, mental, and emotional states are all taken into account before treatment starts.

Reflexologists will assess all the common problems contributing to a patient's ill-health, but their main concern is to establish whether there are any energy imbalances in the zonal pathways. By working and stimulating the reflex that corresponds to the presenting problem, pain relief is often felt, even though the reflex may be far from the particular organ or body part in question. Like acupuncturists, reflexologists believe that by working the reflexes, endorphins will be released, bringing a balance of inner life forces and encouraging the body's innate ability to heal itself.

BELOW *Nutritionally deficient food should be avoided. We need to eat well to feel well.*

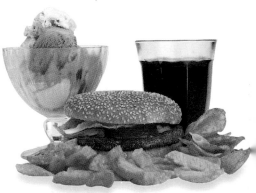

Musculoskeletal Problems

REFLEXOLOGY IS A POWERFUL pain remover in both muscular and skeletal conditions. Toxic build-up may cause rheumatic ache and pains, but this, too, can be helped greatly by reflexology. Other problems that can be helped include fibromyalgia, repetitive strain injury, and frozen shoulder. Bad postural habits are one of the main culprits of back and other skeletal problems, and these should be addressed carefully.

Areas to work

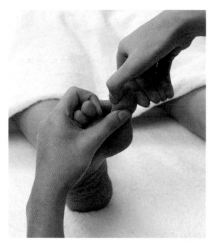

CERVICAL REFLEX

Work the cervical and chronic neck points for neck problems.

NECK REFLEX

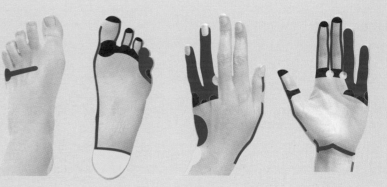

MUSCULOSKELETAL REFLEXES

Individual reflex points are detailed on the charts in Appendix One (pp.130–35).

On the head, the Governor Vessel point GV-26 (in the depression under the nose) will help to strengthen the spine.

DIET

Certain foods can alleviate or aggravate joint inflammation. Fish oils help, while other vegetable oils can aggravate ailments. Ginger will help to relieve rheumatic swelling. Foods that are known to worsen joint pain include wheat and corn cereals, milk, and meat.

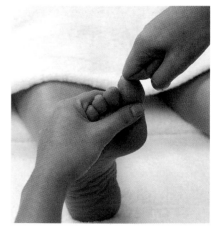

BRAIN REFLEX

Working the brain reflex on the great toe also helps pain, stimulating release of the morphiate-like endorphins (see p. 23).

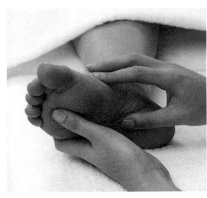

SP-3 POINT

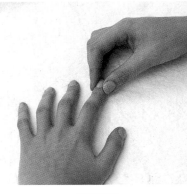

LI-1 POINT

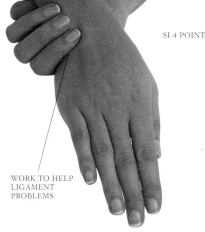

SI-4 POINT

WORK TO HELP
LIGAMENT
PROBLEMS

On the legs, the Spleen meridian point SP-3 (at the lower end of the first joint of the metatarsals – the inner arch at the front of the foot) strengthens the spine. The first Kidney point, KI-1 (in the crease in the middle of the ball of the foot), will relieve lumbago.

On the hands, use the Large Intestine point LI-1 (at the nail bed of the index finger, thumb side) for neck problems.

Use SI-4 and the Heart point HE-4 to aid tendon and ligament problems in the wrist and forearm.

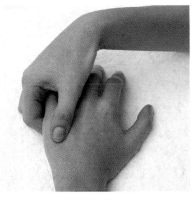

SI-3 POINT

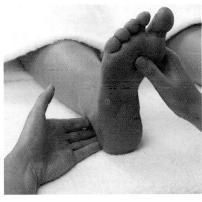

BL-60 POINT

The Bladder point BL-60 (around the lateral ankle bone) is good for severe neck and lumbar pain.

For back problems, use Small Intestine points SI-3 (beneath the little finger, outer edge), SI-4 (at the base of the fifth hand bone), and SI-5 (in the hollow of the wrist joint), which will also relieve problems associated with the knee.

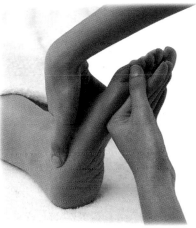

KNEE REFLEX

The knee and elbow reflex can be worked on in any comfortable position. If the person is standing, it can be accessed quite easily.

For back problems, work the spinal reflex on the inner foot and any corresponding muscle area on the outer edge. For knee, leg, hip, or shoulder problems, work the appropriate reflex areas (see p. 55).

Work the adrenal reflexes for rheumatic pain (see p. 51).

(see p. 55). (see p. 51).

CAUTION

Do not use BL-60 in pregnancy, since this point is used for placental retention.

!

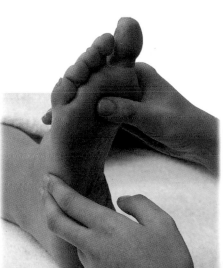

KNEE/ELBOW REFLEX

Nervous Problems

DISORDERS CONNECTED *to the nervous system include painful conditions such as sciatica (radiating lower back pain) and neuralgia (nerve pain), stress-related conditions including insomnia, nervous debility, and depression, and some throat problems (e.g., hoarseness, stuttering); some degenerative conditions (such as Parkinson's disease, Alzheimer's disease, and multiple sclerosis); epilepsy; and some mental problems. Major changes in our lives can create worry and emotional, stress-related disorders; this can lead to many of the so-called "psychosomatic disorders," which can cause a variety of physical symptoms. These range from internal disorders such as high blood pressure, increased heart rate, and poor digestion to muscular pain. All of these symptoms reveal an upset of the internal homeostatic balance. Treatment over a period of time may clear up the causative disorder as well as the symptoms.*

Ailments of the mind can have a devastating effect on the body. Negative thoughts and actions can affect our nervous system, creating nervous disorders. Often the actual cause is exhaustion, worry, or extreme mental strain. When suffering from a nervous disability, many patients complain of a loss of energy, and may feel excess anxiety for no apparent reason, or feelings of despair because they think no one understands them. If the person does not sleep well, then additional irritating symptoms can arise, such as indigestion, constipation, headaches, and irregularities in the female menstrual cycle. The orthodox way of treatment would be antidepressants, sleeping pills, or other tranquilizers. However, this only deadens the pain and does not correct the true cause of the problem. On the other hand,

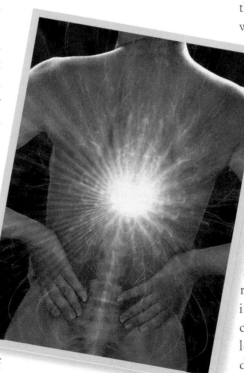

ABOVE *The effects of stress in our lives can cause many psychosomatic illnesses, including muscular pain.*

the natural treatment of reflexology will work on the chemistry of the nervous system, which in time may cause a normalizing of both enzyme and endocrine function.

Blockages within a zonal pathway may overconcentrate the energy in this area, causing a functional nervous imbalance. Such an imbalance may, for instance, occur in either the levels or the balance of various neurotransmitters (*see p. 22*). This imbalance can in turn trigger a response in a muscle or gland. For instance, Parkinson's disease is caused by an imbalance in the levels of the neurotransmitter dopamine; it leads to excess production of a chemical called acetylcholine that is widely used throughout the body, and its visible result is a state that is similar to anxiety, including muscle tremors.

NERVOUS REFLEXES

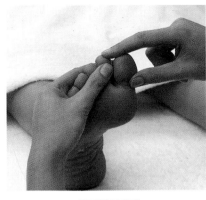

BRAIN REFLEX

SHENMEN POINT

Individual reflex points
are detailed on the charts in
Appendix One (pp.130–35).

Areas to work

*The brain area is contacted when
working on the fingers, toes, or ears.
Work all spine and brain reflexes on
hands and feet, as this will calm the
nerve pathways and balance the
brain chemicals. Such stimulation
also balances the autonomic nervous
system (see p. 20).*

*(ii) Of particular note for calming the
mind is the Shenmen point (HE-7, on
the little-finger side of the wrist
crease). Half a thumb's-width up from
this is another Heart meridian point
used for insomnia (HE-6).*

PE-6 POINT

*(iii) The Pericardium
meridian runs down
the middle of the
inner forearm. Two
points lying two and
three thumb-widths up
from the wrist crease
(PE-6 and 5), and the
terminal point at the
tip of the second finger
(PE-9), may all be used
for depression.*

SHIXUAN POINT

PRESS TIPS
OF FINGERS

SHIXUAN POINT

*On the hand
and forearm,
several points are
beneficial.
(i) Pressure on the tips
of the fingers, known
in T.C.M. as the
"Shixuan" points, helps
in acute problems.
(Remember, the hands
occupy a large sensory
area in the brain, so the
tips are extremely sensitive
to pressure.)*

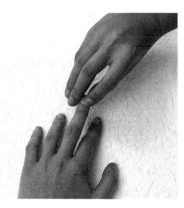

PE-9 POINT

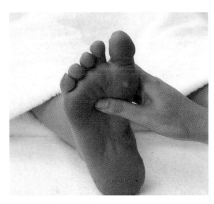

KI-1 POINT

On the foot, the first Kidney point (KI-1, in the crease behind the ball of the foot), is a major point for its tranquilizing effect, is beneficial for insomnia, and is a wonderful balancing point.

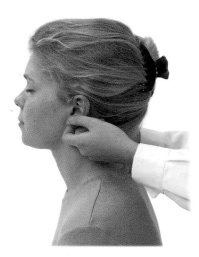

SUBCORTEX POINT

(ii) A point on the lower cartilage projection is also used for depression as it has pain-relieving qualities for the nervous system.

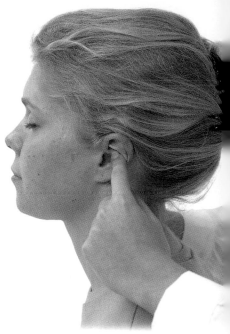

ZERO POINT

(iii) For insomnia, the center of the ear is used to contact the vagus nerve (see p. 63), slowing the heart rate.

TIP

As well as regular reflexology treatments, try to include plenty of carbohydrates in your diet to help calm and soothe the nerves.

STROKE TO
RELIEVE
DEPRESSION

Points used on the ear are as follows:

(i) Stroking the ears will relieve both depression and insomnia.

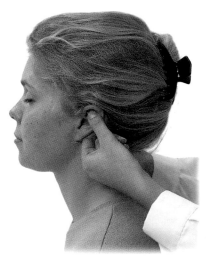

SCIATIC NERVE POINT

(iv) A point on the antihelix is specific for sciatica. The sciatic nerve is a major nerve of the leg. Problems can effect the lumbar and sacral areas. Pressure on this point will relieve pain and any persistent weakness or numbness.

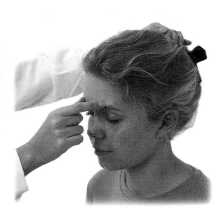

BL-2 POINT

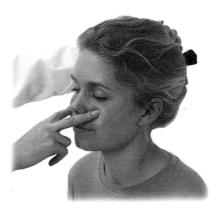

ST-1 POINT

Several points on the head will help neurological problems.
(i) For pain in the jaw and cheek area (trigeminal neuralgia), use any of these points: on the midline (GB-14) or the medial edges (BL-2) of the eyebrow, the points between the eyebrow and the ear, the first Stomach meridian points (ST-1 and 2) just below the eyes, or the Large Intestine points (LI-20) by the base of the nose.

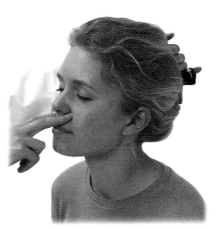

L1-20 POINT

DIET

Include the herb parsley in your diet, as it helps to stimulate activity in the brain. A couple of cups of coffee can also have a stimulating effect on the nervous system, but there are adverse effects from excess caffeine (from tea, coffee, and some soda drinks), as a high intake is thought to irritate nerves, creating jumpiness. Protein-rich foods also have a stimulating effect on brain activity, as they help prevent a buildup of the neurotransmitter serotonin, a sleep-inducing chemical that tends to make you drowsy (*see Hormones and Neurotransmitters, pp. 22–23*). Foods containing the trace mineral boron – including nuts, leafy vegetables, legumes, and some fruits, such as apples – also aid mental alertness. To lift your mood, eat foods rich in folic acid (such as green leafy vegetables), selenium (seafood, brazil nuts), and carbohydrates.

GV-16 POINT

GOOD FOR MENTAL PROBLEMS

GV-16 POINT

(ii) For epilepsy and mental problems, a good point is on the Governor Vessel (GV-16), on the hairline in the midline of the body.

SPINAL REFLEX

The spinal reflex can be worked around the outside edge of the thumb and palm.

STRESS

Stress is defined as any stimulus or factor that threatens the health of the body or has an adverse effect on its functioning. Extreme stress (for example, wounds from accidents) can cause great changes in the body, such as a drastic drop in blood pressure, precipitating circulatory collapse. In these acute cases, Western medicine can be most beneficial. However, medication can help the symptoms of stress, but it will not cure the problem until you remove the causative factors. Even mild stress can be a contributory factor in conditions such as ulcers, migraines, heart attacks, eczema, diabetes, and even cancer.

People vary in the amount of stress they are able to tolerate, but eventually stress overstimulates the adrenal gland. This controls the way our physical and mental systems respond to threat or challenge. Two substances that are produced by the adrenal glands – epinephrine (adrenaline) and norepinephrine (noradrenaline) – are released in response to short bursts of activity

BELOW *In cases of extreme stress, such as in accidents, the body changes are severe and life-threatening.*

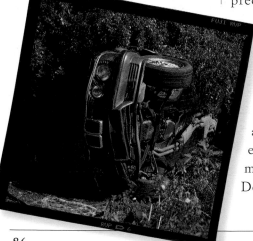

THE EFFECTS OF STRESS ON THE BODY

- heart rate quickens

- breathing becomes deeper and faster

- blood flow to the muscles increases

- blood sugar level rises to release more energy

- increased alertness triggers emotional reactions

or stress, and they prepare the body physiologically for "fight or flight," increasing the heart rate, diverting blood from the digestive organs to the muscles, increasing alertness, and triggering emotional reactions. However, adrenal stimulation over a long period will deplete the body's systems. This is often also because of insufficient exercise and relaxation, as the excess amount of epinephrine is not metabolized. Constant stress can also change hormone balance.

Chronic stress can be caused by long-term emotional problems. Pressure in everyday life can cause biochemical changes in the body, precipitating such conditions as headaches or lower back problems. Indirectly, this may also contribute to high blood pressure, digestive disorders, anxiety, and depression. To some degree, everyone feels sad at some time or another, and even the most successful people may suffer from anxiety at times. Depression can be a passing

phase; but it can also become a long-term burden in which the person is prone to frequent inner emptiness and despair, while acute depression is often the result of bereavement or a failed relationship.

Reflexology cannot remove the stress, but it can help the stress responses that may arise. It is relaxing, giving an inner tranquility, which helps you to cope better with stressful situations. It also helps many of the physical symptoms that may have arisen, balancing the whole biological system on which our health depends.

It is important to learn how to relax properly. It is not enough to sit in front of the television after work, as this does not completely relax you. If you look around, you will find there are many different methods of relaxation available, from yoga, Tai Chi, qigong, or meditation, to books or tapes on relaxation techniques. It is worthwhile putting in time and practice to become a cool, calm, and collected person, as relaxation is a prerequisite to achieving health.

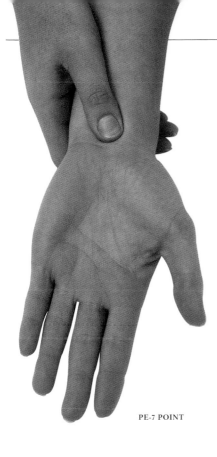

PE-7 POINT

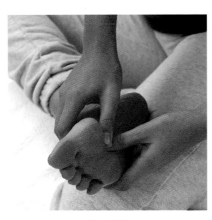

KI-1 POINT

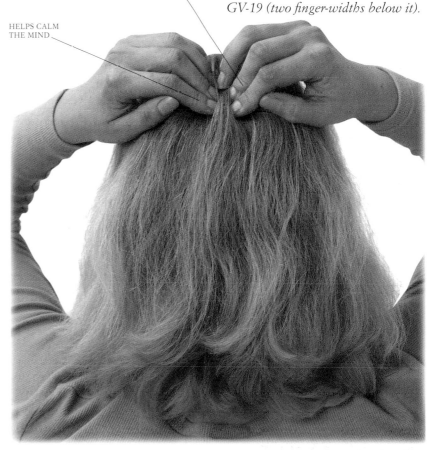

GV-20 POINT

On the feet, the first Kidney meridian point (KI-1, in the crease of the sole of the foot just behind the ball of the foot) is a major T.C.M. point for relaxation.

Points on the head useful for calming the mind include the middle of the eyebrows, and two points on the Governor Vessel, running down the midline – the Baihui point GV-20 (on a line connecting the ears over the top of the head), and the point GV-19 (two finger-widths below it).

GV-19 POINT

HELPS CALM THE MIND

Areas to work

Stroke around the palmar (inside) surface of the wrists, from the little-finger edge to the thumb edge. There are three acupoints located on the wrist crease that aid relaxation, and which are also stress-calming points. These are the Heart meridian point HE-7 (on the little-finger side), the Pericardium point PE-7 (on the inner forearm), and the Lung point LU-9 (on the thumb side).

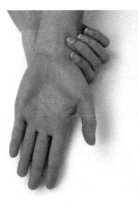

LU-9 POINT

GV-19 POINT

DIET

To alleviate stress and anxiety, include more complex carbohydrates such as pasta, cereals, legumes, and vegetables in your diet; these are believed to encourage the amino acid tryptophan to enter the brain, where it is converted to serotonin, the neurotransmitter (*see p. 23*) that has a calming effect. For a faster-acting tranquilizing effect, drink a noncaffeine drink containing honey to induce relaxation and drowsiness. Onions contain a mild sedative called quercetin, which acts on the central nervous system.

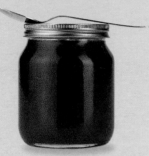

HONEY

ABOVE AND BELOW *To alleviate stress, include plenty of fresh vegetables and complex carbohydrates in your diet; honey in a noncaffeine drink is a great mind soother.*

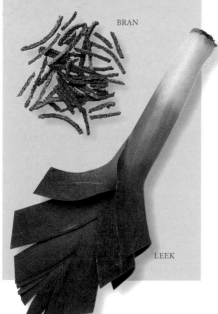

BRAN

LEEK

VISUALIZATION

In your imagination, try to visualize your own ideal stress-free situation and then concentrate on this image for at least three or four minutes. For instance, you might visualize an open window through which all your problems are passing, or you may imagine you are a bird flying away from everything stressful in your life. You may like to imagine yourself relaxing on a beach with the water lapping around your feet, or you could try to imagine that you are floating on a cloud. Use any other image that gives you a personal sense of peace and well-being.

CONCENTRATE FOR A FEW MINUTES ON A STRESS-FREE IMAGE

FEEL THE INNER CALM

BREATHE IN THROUGH YOUR NOSE

SIMPLE BREATHING EXERCISES

There are many variations of these. The following is one of the simplest. Ideally, lie flat on the floor, although this can also be practiced sitting in a comfortable position. Breathe in through your nose, slowly and deeply, for three counts. Hold your breath for three counts. Then breathe out slowly through your mouth for three counts. Continue from the beginning, keeping a steady rhythm, for three or four minutes. As you breathe, and particularly as you hold your breath, make sure your muscles are relaxed.

You can repeat the above, this time holding a finger on one nostril. Then change and do the other nostril, so that you are breathing first through one and then the other.

EXERCISES TO RELIEVE STRESS

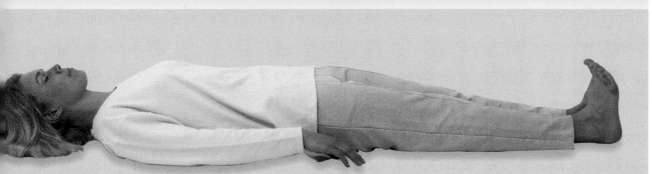

PROGRESSIVE MUSCULAR RELAXATION

The aim of this is to work through each of the main groups of muscles in the body, first tensing and then relaxing each in turn.

Lie on your back on the floor, with your arms by your sides, and your feet uncrossed. Starting with your toes and feet, tense and hold these muscles for a few seconds, then slowly relax them. Repeat this exercise with your calf muscles, thighs, buttocks, back (arch gently and relax), stomach, arms and shoulders, and face (the mouth, nose, eyes, and forehead, each in turn). Finish with the deep-breathing exercise on p.88.

REFLEXOLOGY RELAXATION TECHNIQUES

Practice with your fingers first. Tense and hold them for five seconds and then relax, allowing the sense of relaxation to travel up your arms and into your shoulders. Breathe deeply. Repeat this with your toes. Rotate your wrist and then your ankles. Stretch them and then relax. Clasp your hands together and hold for a few minutes.

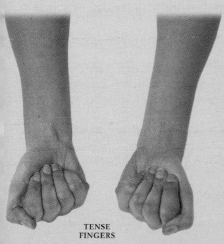

TENSE FINGERS

CLASP HANDS

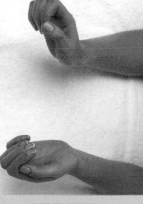

HOLD HANDS TOGETHER FOR A FEW MINUTES

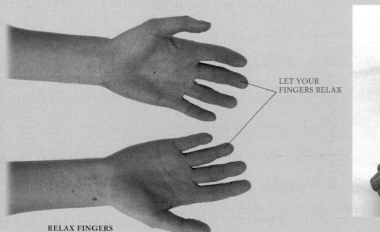

LET YOUR FINGERS RELAX

RELAX FINGERS

ROTATE WRISTS

Head and Neck Problems

HEADACHES *are a common problem that may be diffuse or one-sided, as in migraines. Other problems in this area include ear and hearing problems, eye disorders, nose problems, and neck stiffness.*

MIGRAINES AND OTHER HEADACHES

A migraine is an intense headache that can be caused by a variety of triggers, such as anxiety, tiredness, certain foods, and hormonal imbalances. In a classical migraine, there is often accompanying sickness or a blurring of vision, but many lesser forms also occur. Other headaches may be related to anxiety (*see pp. 82–87*), overuse of the eyes, or digestive imbalance. Reflexology aids in relaxing constricted blood vessels, and in calming. Treatment over a period of time can help to alleviate the disorder completely.

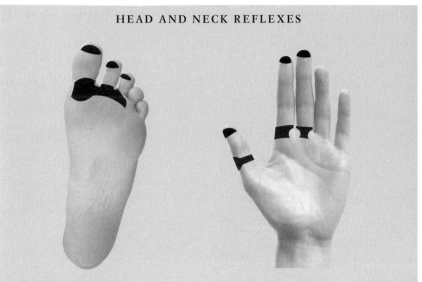

HEAD AND NECK REFLEXES

Individual reflex points are detailed on the charts in Appendix One (pp.130–35).

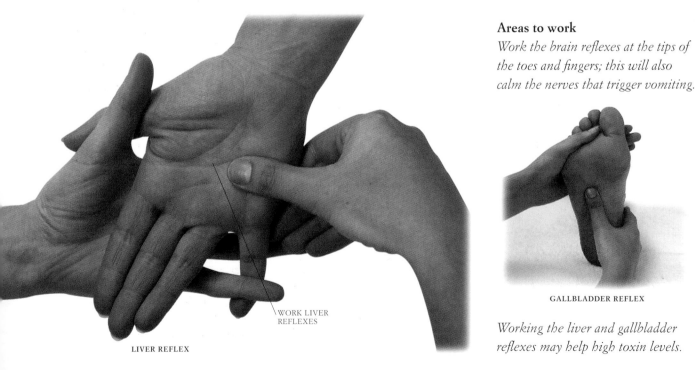

WORK LIVER REFLEXES

LIVER REFLEX

Areas to work
Work the brain reflexes at the tips of the toes and fingers; this will also calm the nerves that trigger vomiting.

GALLBLADDER REFLEX

Working the liver and gallbladder reflexes may help high toxin levels.

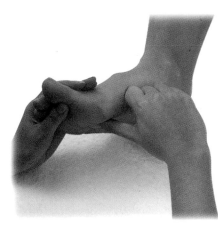

SPINAL REFLEX

Use your knuckles to sweep up and down the the spinal reflex on the feet; this calms the whole central nervous system.

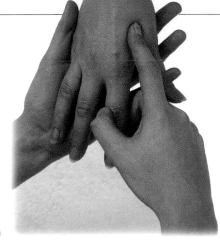

LI-4 POINT

The Large Intestine point LI-4 (in the web of the thumb and index finger) gives extra pain relief, particularly where there is facial neuralgia.

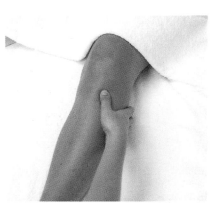

ST-36 POINT

On the leg, the Stomach meridian point ST-36 (four finger-widths below the kneecap) relieves digestive, frontal headaches.

On the ear, the Shenmen point (in the triangular fossa depression) will give pain relief and have a calming action on the mind.

On the head and neck are a number of points that relieve headaches:
(i) The points on each temple one thumb's-width behind the eyebrow edge are good for migraines.
(ii) The point midway between the eyebrows may be used for headaches.
(iii) The Baihui point GV-20 (at the crown of the head) is particularly calming for stress-induced headaches. The adjacent point (GV-19, two finger-widths below it) is also indicated for migraines (see p. 71).

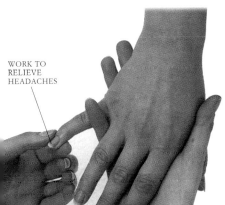

WORK TO RELIEVE HEADACHES

SI-1 POINT

On the hand, there are two acupoints that will help:
The first point on the Small Intestine meridian (SI-1, on the outside edge of the nail bed on the little finger) helps to relieve headaches generally.

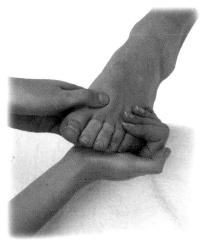

LIV-3 POINT

On the foot, the Liver meridian point LIV-3 (in the furrow between the first and second toes) helps migraine and digestive headaches.

CAUTION

Do not use ST-36 on young children. The LI-4 point must not be used during pregnancy.

DIET

Many foods contain chemicals that trigger headaches in genetically susceptible people by initiating neural and blood vessel changes. The most common triggers are drinks containing caffeine, chocolate, mature cheese, cured meats, alcohol (especially red wine), monosodium glutamate, salt, and nuts. Foods that will help to relieve headaches include oily fish, fish oils, and ginger, which acts in a similar way to aspirin to combat the inflammation.

NECK PROBLEMS

These include pain or stiffness when turning the neck. This can result from problems with the cervical (neck) vertebrae themselves, or from injury or disease to the peripheral nerves supplying the neck. Incorrect posture may also be a contributory factor in neck problems.

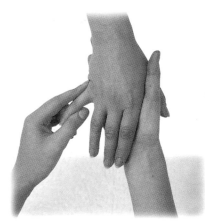

CERVICAL REFLEX

Points to use
Work the cervical reflex and the chronic neck points.

On the hands, use the first Small Intestine points SI-1 (see p.91), SI-2 (at the base of the little finger, outside edge), and SI-3 (on the outside edge of the hand, by the knuckle), or the first Large Intestine point LI-1 (at the nail bed of the index finger, thumb-side).

The Bladder point BL-10 and the Gallbladder point GB-20 ("Fengchi") may be used for neck stiffness and pain.

WORK AT THE
NAIL BED ON
INDEX FINGER

LI-1 POINT

EAR PROBLEMS

Ear problems should never be neglected. Earaches are often caused by infection; this travels from the nose, throat, or teeth. A weeping inflammation called *otitis media* is common in young children. Treatment aims to relieve the congested state by breaking down excess mucus or catarrh. (*See p. 62.*)

Areas to work
Start by working the ear points, facial points, and head-related areas. Also work the upper cervical reflex, as this connects with the vagus nerve (see p. 63), which serves the ear. Work the adrenal reflex to alleviate inflammation.

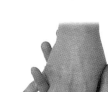

EAR REFLEXES

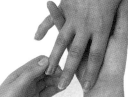

TB-1 POINT

On the hands, use the Triple Burner points TB-1 (at the base of the third fingernail bed) and TB-2 (in the web between the third and fourth fingers).

On the head, the point in the depression next to the ear is the last point on the Small Intestine meridian (SI-19); it is useful for all ear disorders, including ringing in the ears, weeping inflammation, and deafness.

LI-1 POINT

EYE PROBLEMS

Most general eye disorders can be helped enormously with reflexology. The majority of minor inflammations, such as conjunctivitis, can be greatly eased. With aging, other problems, such as cataracts, can occur; even regular medication can create an imbalance within the eyes. Any sudden change in vision should always be investigated; however, there are many points that can be worked to aid everyday problems.

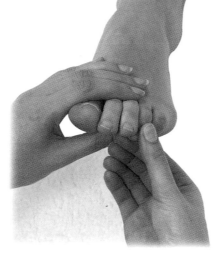

GB-44 POINT

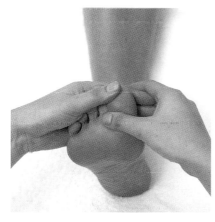

CERVICAL REFLEXES

Areas to work

Work the eye reflexes on the digits in zones 2 to 3. The neck reflexes stimulate the nerve pathways, and the brain reflex stimulates the optic nerve. The kidneys also have a zonal link to the eyes. Work the adrenal reflex to alleviate inflammation.

On the legs, the Gallbladder points GB-44 (on the nail bed of the fourth toe, outside edge) is for any eye disorder, while GB-37 (five thumbwidths above the outside ankle bone on the side of the lower leg, in front of the fibula bone) is known as "eye bright," as it prevents eye degeneration.

On the head, the following points relate to the eyes. The first and second Bladder points, BL-1 (just above the inner corner of each eye) and BL-2 (on the inner edge of each eyebrow), are useful for treating conjunctivitis, near-sightedness, "floaters" in the eyes, and glaucoma. The points in the middle of each eyebrow are for conjunctivitis and brightening the eyes. The first Gallbladder point, GB-1 (on the outer corner of the eye), the Triple Burner point TB-23 (on the outer edge of the eyebrow), and the first Stomach point, ST-1 (on the the bone just below the center of the eye), may also be used. You can apply pressure to each of the above points in turn.

NASAL PROBLEMS

Many nasal problems may be aided by reflexology, including sinusitis and inflammation of the nasal membranes, which may be caused by allergy or infection.

Points to use

Work the reflexes to the nose (below) and facial areas. Work the adrenal reflex to alleviate inflammation.

On the head, the point midway between the eyebrows and that in the depression under the nose (LI-20, the last Large Intestine point) are useful (see pp. 69 and 139). The latter is indicated for nosebleeds, loss of the sense of smell, and allergic rhinitis (inflammation).

NASAL REFLEXES

NASAL REFLEX

Respiratory Problems

RESPIRATORY DISORDERS include coughs, colds, bronchitis, emphysema (a pathologic accumulation of air in the lungs, leading to breathing difficulties), and asthma, or any conditions involving congestion or inflammation of the lungs or respiratory passages. They are often associated with smoking, climatic conditions, or pollution, or the cause may be a bacterial or viral infection, such as a cold. The exact causes of asthma are still being debated, but there is commonly a strong association with stress.

The following self-help tips are for all sufferers with respiratory problems. However, many people will benefit from regular professional treatments, because as we age our lungs tend to lose their natural elasticity, so regular reflexology treatment enables the respiratory process to function better.

ASTHMA

Asthma is caused by a hyper-sensitivity to stimuli on the lining of the bronchial tubes in the lungs (*see p. 48*). This results in a narrowing of these and the nasal passages owing to thickening, inflammation, and excess mucus production, as well as excessive muscular contractions, causing spasms. The sufferer can usually inhale air into the lungs, but is unable to exhale fully and may also wheeze as a result of restriction of the windpipe or bronchial tubes. The usual medical treatment is the use of a bronchodilator in the form of an inhaler; in severe cases, corticosteroids (steroids) are used to reduce the inflammation. However, persistent use of these medications can cause hoarseness, and high doses can affect the heart rate and sometimes induce fine muscular tremors, headaches, and nervous tension. Corticosteroids will also act to reduce the body's natural immune response.

Reflexology can aid an asthmatic person by allowing freer and easier breathing and removing tension in the diaphragm area. (*See also Bronchitis, p.96*)

CAUTION
Reflexology should not be used instead of professional medical advice; for any acute breathlessness see a physician immediately.

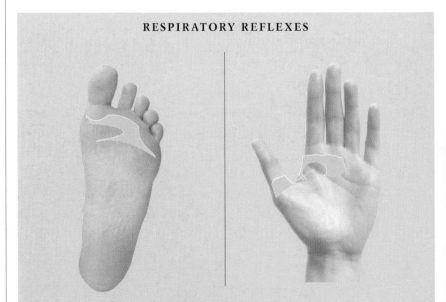

RESPIRATORY REFLEXES

Individual reflex points are detailed on the charts in Appendix One (pp.130–35).

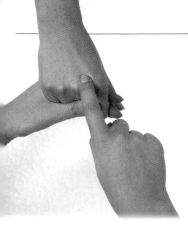

LUNG REFLEX

Areas to work

Start by working the lung reflex area on either hands or feet. On the hands, this is on the pads of the palm below the fingers; on the feet, it is on the ball of the foot.

On the hands, the reflex points are a powerful and energetic area to work in this condition. These reflexes can be worked daily without any undue side effects, and great benefit can be obtained from them.

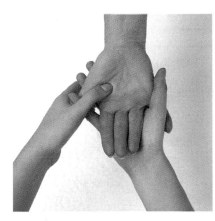

ADRENAL GLAND REFLEX

Also, work any of the adrenal points. The adrenal gland reflex can be found in the hand on the base of the web between the thumb and index finger on the palmar surface only. On the feet, it lies in the upper arch on the inner edge.

On the hands, two acupoints are particularly useful:
(i) The first point is the Large Intestine point LI-4 (in the web between the thumb and index finger). It is a general point for relief of nasal and breathing problems, such as allergic rhinitis (nasal inflammation), hayfever, sneezing, and runny, itchy eyes; it also has a stimulating but dispersing effect on the lungs.
(ii) The second point is a Lung meridian point (LU-11, on the thumb, on the outside corner of the nail bed). Continue to press all around the thumb, down to the fleshy prominent part at the base, then down to the wrist area for about 3 inches; this will aid removal of phlegm and excess mucus.

DIET

Most asthmatics and other people with breathing problems produce excess mucus, and they need to be aware of certain foods that can aggravate this. Dairy products such as milk, cheese, butter, and chocolate all increase mucus levels. Smoking, and drinking alcohol, particularly at night, irritate and swell the mucous membrane lining the throat, which may impair the air flow to the lungs. Garlic aids in bronchial congestion.

On the legs is another point, on the Stomach meridian (ST-40, which lies six finger-widths below the knee in between the tibia and fibula bones). Pressure applied here will help to eliminate phlegm.

On the ear, a point on the cartilage projection above the lobe will alleviate asthma.

LU-11 POINT

WORK TO REMOVE PHLEGM AND EXCESS MUCUS

CAUTION
Do not use LI-4 in pregnancy.
!

LU-11

RESPIRATORY INFECTIONS

In these conditions, there is generally a narrowing of the bronchial passageways as a result of congestion. Respiratory conditions can cause problems at different levels of the respiratory tract, inflaming the larynx (laryngitis), pharynx (pharyngitis), or bronchial tubes (bronchitis). Tension or anxiety further diminishes the ability of the lungs to take in sufficient oxygen; tension on the diaphragm muscle frequently causes it to go into spasm, so the lungs cannot expand enough. Regular reflexology treatment acts as a counterirritant, relieving deep-seated discomfort by relaxing the bronchial muscles.

SPINAL AND CERVICAL REFLEXES

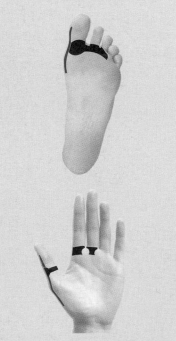

Individual reflex points are detailed on the charts in Appendix One (pp.130–35).

Areas to work

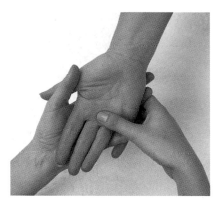

CERVICAL REFLEX

Work the spinal and cervical reflexes to stimulate the smooth bronchial muscles and the phrenic nerve in the neck area, which runs to the diaphragm and membranes surrounding the lung; this helps to insure regular contractions of the diaphragm during breathing.

The hands are a marvelous area to use. Work as for asthma. Press all over the brain reflex on the great toe and thumb, at the tips and the base of the digits, to help facilitate the breathing process and stimulate the vagus nerve (see p. 63) *to slow the breathing and heart rate.*

On the hands, the Large Intestine point LI-4 (in the web of the thumb and first finger) helps all head-related areas and relieves many cold symptoms.

DIET

Eat garlic, known as "nature's antibiotic," as it has both antibacterial and antiviral properties. It is generally beneficial to the respiratory tract, aiding the mucous membranes and purifying the blood. Leeks and onions have similar properties, and also aid the breakup of phlegm, as do hot spices such as mustard, ginger, and chilis. For viral infections, you need to drink lots of (preferably hot) liquids; a traditional Chinese remedy is hot chicken soup. If you have a tendency toward bronchitis, insure you include plenty of vitamin C in your diet.

On the ear, the following points help: (i) The six points on the helix are for all upper respiratory infections (see p. 64). *(ii) Stroking the back of the ear close to the crease contacts two points. The first is the point contacting the vagus nerve directly; this has an immediate effect on the organs of the chest cavity. The second is the lung point next to it.*

WORK THE HELIX POINTS FOR RESPIRATORY INFECTIONS

HELIX POINTS

EXERCISES FOR ASTHMA

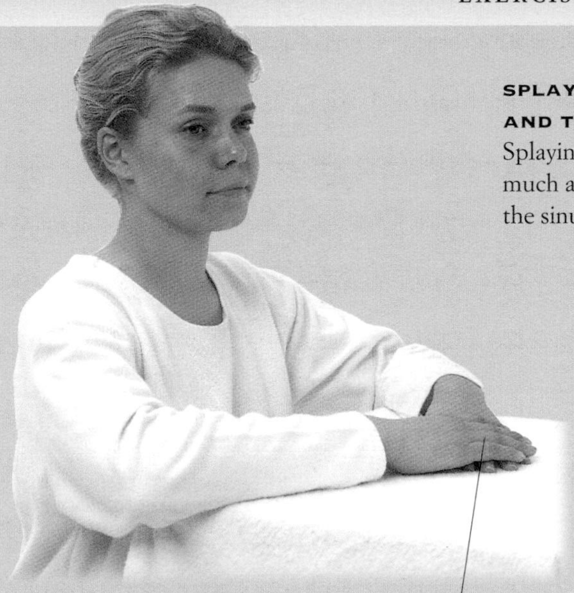

SPLAYING FINGERS AND TOES

Splaying fingers and toes as much as possible (this helps the sinuses).

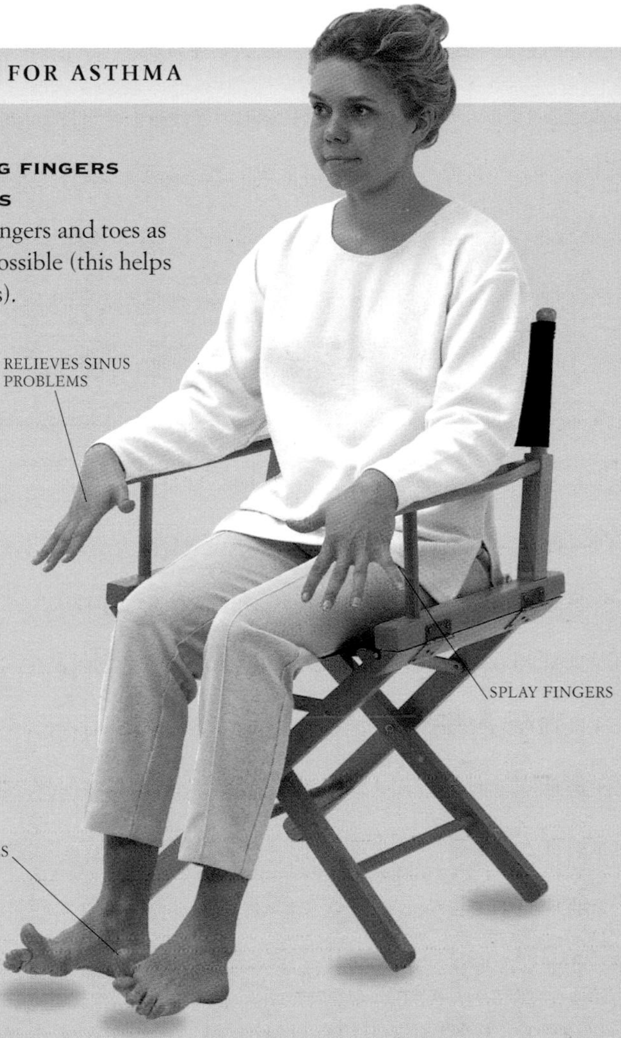

RELIEVES SINUS PROBLEMS

SPLAY FINGERS

SPLAY TOES

REST HANDS ON SUPPORT

RAISING ELBOWS

A good exercise is to raise the elbows almost to shoulder level, resting them on a support while leaning forward; this exercise lifts the diaphragm, which helps in exhalation. Also, stand on the tips of the toes; this will apply pressure on the ball of the foot (the lung area).

PRESSING PALMS

Press the upper palms of the hands together (the lung area).

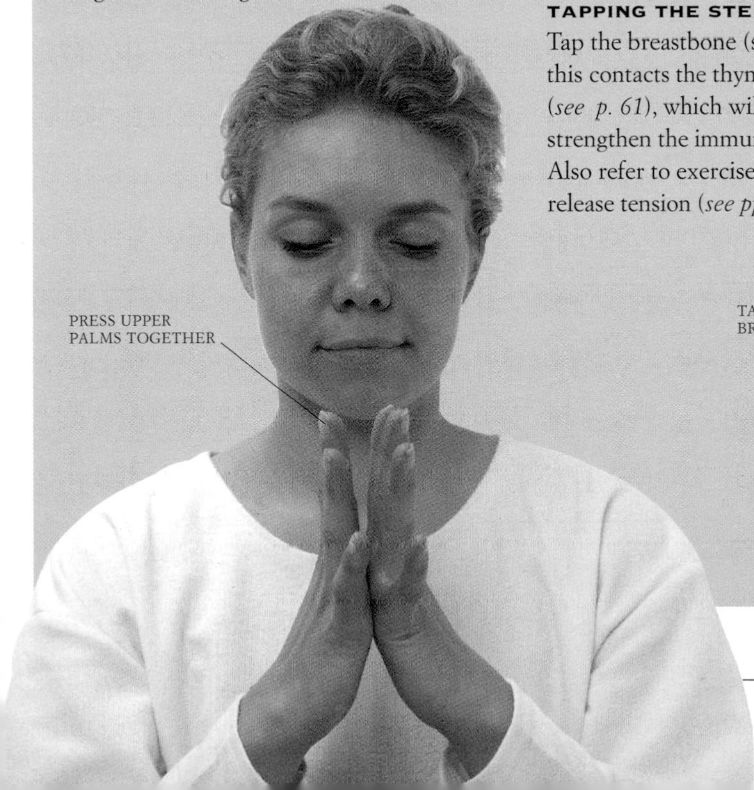

TAPPING THE STERNUM

Tap the breastbone (sternum); this contacts the thymus gland (*see p. 61*), which will strengthen the immune system. Also refer to exercises to release tension (*see pp. 88–89*).

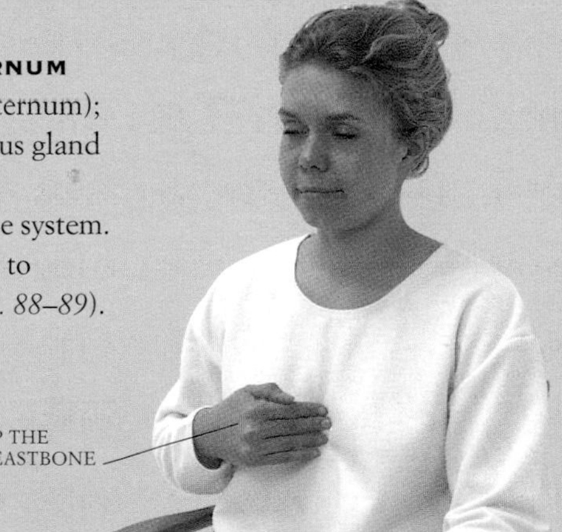

TAP THE BREASTBONE

PRESS UPPER PALMS TOGETHER

97

Digestive and Bowel Problems

WHEN WE THINK *how the alimentary canal has to deal with some of the food we eat, which is often in excess to our needs, we can see why there is such a great prevalence of diseases of the gastrointestinal tract and bowels. These disorders often manifest themselves in stressful situations, when eating too quickly, or when angry. Reflexology achieves the necessary relaxation that aids and influences the course of digestion. Working the reflex points that stimulate the vagus nerve (see p. 63) heightens the activity of the parasympathetic nervous system and therefore stimulates the digestive processes, and the nerves and muscles of the gut wall, so the proper peristaltic rhythm is maintained to propel food along the gut.*

INDIGESTION AND GASTRIC DISORDERS

Indigestion is an all-embracing word for many digestive discomforts, from swelling and distension of the stomach to ulceration. Many painful and uncomfortable problems such as acid or nervous dyspepsia (discomfort of the stomach after meals), catarrh of the stomach, or even intestinal spasm, are relieved with treatment.

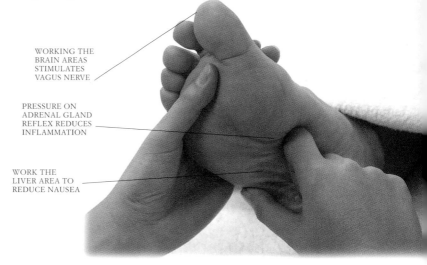

WORKING THE BRAIN AREAS STIMULATES VAGUS NERVE

PRESSURE ON ADRENAL GLAND REFLEX REDUCES INFLAMMATION

WORK THE LIVER AREA TO REDUCE NAUSEA

ADRENAL GLAND REFLEX

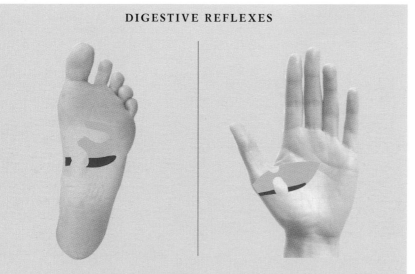

DIGESTIVE REFLEXES

Individual reflex points are detailed on the charts in Appendix One (pp.130–35).

Areas to work

The main reflex area to work is that corresponding to the organ where the primary problem is felt, between the ball and the heel area of the soles of the feet. Extra pressure on the adrenal gland reflex will reduce inflammation. Where there is biliousness, work the liver and gallbladder reflexes on the right foot or hand. On the left foot the stomach and pancreas. Stimulate the vagus nerve, which increases salivation and gastric secretions, by pressing the brain area on the great toe.

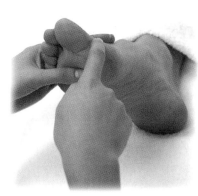

SP-2 POINT

On the lower legs, the Spleen meridian point SP-2 (in the middle of the lower bone on the great toe) aids digestion. On the front surface, the Stomach points ST-35 (beside the kneecap), ST-36 (four finger-widths below the knee, outside the tibia bone), and ST-39 (in the middle of the lower leg) will regulate the stomach's activity, and can relieve inflammation (gastritis).

CAUTION

ST-36 should not be used on young children.

TB-6 POINT

STIMULATES FOOD
ELIMINATION

On the arms, the Triple Burner points TB-3 (on the back of the hand, between the bones on a line between the ring and little fingers), TB-4 and TB-6 (on the same line above the flexure of the wrist). These points stimulate food elimination and aid constipation. The Large Intestine point LI-3 (at the base of the first finger, inner edge) relieves flatulence.

DIET

Many different foods can aggravate or help digestive disorders. For ulcers, although a bacterial infection is now considered a main cause, foods such as milk, beer, and caffeine-containing drinks can be an aggravating factor, while bananas and cabbage juice have beneficial effects. For heartburn, or acid indigestion, cut back on fatty foods and eat more complex carbohydrates, such as vegetables and wholegrain cereals. Chocolate, coffee, alcohol, raw onions, citrus juice, or hot spicy foods may be aggravating the problem. Sufferers from wind may need to cut down on milk, beans, and some vegetables, particularly of the onion or brassica family, while ginger, garlic, and peppermint help to prevent wind. For nausea, ginger is a good dietary aid. Banana also helps to relieve dyspepsia.

On the ear, the center of ear points (back and front) also stimulate the vagus nerve.

CAUTION

In any serious or long-term bowel disorder, it is imperative to have a thorough medical examination for the cause of the problem; it is also advisable to have regular treatments from a professionally qualified practitioner who would adopt a holistic view.

ST-39 POINT
RELIEVES
GASTRITIS

ST-39 POINT

BOWEL DISORDERS

Colonic disorders are now very common; most are due to buildup of waste materials, poor diet, indigestion, or even tension and stress. Abdominal swelling and distension can be caused by inflammation and protusion of body structures through the membrane that lines the intestinal tract (diverticulitis); these create small pouches causing lower abdominal pain, followed by either diarrhea or constipation. Irritable bowel syndrome (colic, constipation, and diarrhea with excess mucus production) is also common; the cause is often unknown. Crohn's disease is a severe irritation of the intestinal tract lining; it can occur in any part of the tract from the mouth to the anus, but often the bowel wall is most affected. It can lead to scarring, thickening, obstruction, anal abscesses or fistulas (an abnormal passage opening up to the surface of the skin). Many sufferers find that diet can aggravate or alleviate the symptoms. Medications can also create constipation.

DIET

Broccoli helps to maintain a healthy intestinal area and also aids elimination. Bananas are rich in potassium; they alleviate the effects of diarrhea, which often causes loss of potassium. This mineral is also an aid in many sporting activities, where excessive sweating takes place; eating a banana will benefit the muscular system and insure that muscle spasm does not occur. Oranges and apples will also help the bowels by stimulating elimination.

Usually, regular treatment with reflexology encourages correct muscular activity of the stomach; it also stimulates the production of the gastric juices and improves peristalsis (see p. 52), controlling the rate of digestion and the speed of passage of food along the digestive tract. Excessive activity in the bowels is stemmed and an overall coordinated activity returns that helps with both constipation and diarrhea.

The following procedures produce a counterirritant effect and stimulate the healing reflex; they can be used in order to relieve any deep-seated pain or discomfort.

Areas to work

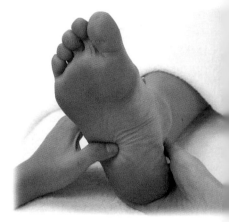

ILEOCECAL VALVE REFLEX

For all sluggish bowel conditions, work on the tips of the toes or fingers for stimulation to the cranial nerves. Stimulation must also be given to the liver/gallbladder area, because bile helps peristalsis in the duodenum. Firm extra pressure on the reflex to the ileocecal valve, which controls the passage of food from the small to the large intestine (see p. 52), *seems to stimulate the strong rhythmic, muscular contractions of the large intestines so that the contents are propelled forward (the contents have to move against gravity). This also insures efficient functioning, as this valve is there to prevent backflow of waste into the small intestines. Use if there is any diarrhea or inflammatory disorder within the mucous membrane or if there is any infection present.*

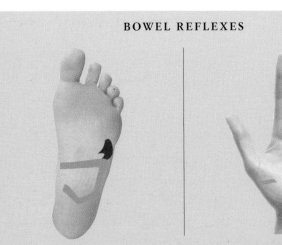

BOWEL REFLEXES

Individual reflex points are detailed on the charts in Appendix One (pp.130–35).

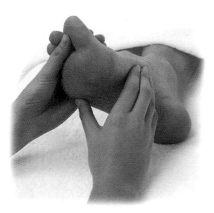

SPINAL REFLEX

THIS POINT
RELATES TO THE
SYMPATHETIC
NERVOUS SYSTEM

HELPS
ABDOMINAL
CRAMPS

CALMS NERVE
SIGNALS TO
BOWEL WALL

Three areas need extra stimulation:
(i) Stimulation to the adrenal gland reflex area encourages the adrenals to produce very powerful anti-inflammatory compounds called glucocorticoids (which include corticosterone and hydrocortisone or cortisol); it also helps the regulation of salt and water balance, alleviating the loss of vital body salts (e.g., potassium), which occurs with excessive diarrhea.

(ii) Stimulation of the spinal area contacts the sympathetic nervous system (see p. 21); *this decreases activity in the bowels and helps to calm the transmission of the nerve signals to the bowel wall.*

(iii) The spleen is a vital area for both of these problems; this organ adjusts the quality and quantity of blood in the circulation and, according to T.C.M., is responsible for peristalsis in the colon. It also helps to remove foreign bodies from the bloodstream. Extra stimulation to this reflex area helps its contraction, thus squeezing every bit of nutrient-rich blood into the general circulation.

ABDOMINAL REFLEX

AIDS DIGESTION

RESPONSIBLE FOR
PERISTALSIS IN
THE COLON

SPLEEN REFLEX

On the ear, the following points are indicated:
(i) On the antihelix is a point relating to the sympathic nervous system; this will help in relieving abdominal cramps.
(ii) In the upper part of the concha is a point used for abdominal swelling.

On the face, the last point on the Conception Vessel (CV-24, on the midline on the lower lip) will relieve constipation.

CAUTION
If there is severe pain, it is imperative to seek medical advice as soon as possible.

CALCULI (STONES)

Stones forming in the gallbladder are caused by a homeostatic imbalance. An imbalance within the gallbladder and bile ducts causes alterations in bile production. Since bile keeps cholesterol more soluble, a drop in its production is one of the major factors in the formation of gallstones in which cholesterol, bile pigments, and calcium salts form a hard mass. Stones can be present for many years, and will create colicky pain of varying levels. However, if stones pass into the bile duct, they then can create a major problem causing the person to suffer excruciating pain symptoms shortly after a meal, and surgery is then needed.

VAGUS NERVE CONTACTS GALLBLADDER REFLEX

WORK THE BIG TOE

VAGUS NERVE STIMULATES GALLBLADDER

DIET

A low fat diet is essential. Cutting out all dairy products, drinking fresh lemon juice in hot water, or taking a teaspoonful of pure olive oil daily are beneficial. Celery in any form aids in elimination and is an alkaline vegetable that is purported to be beneficial for any overacidity. Dandelion tea is an age-old remedy as a liver cleanser and for stimulating bile production.

Areas to work

With reflexology, you can balance the system by working the liver and gallbladder reflexes directly. Working the great toe or thumb (and stroking behind the ear) will contact the vagus nerve (see p. 63); this nerve stimulates both the liver and the gallbladder, which in turn stimulate the secretion of bile.

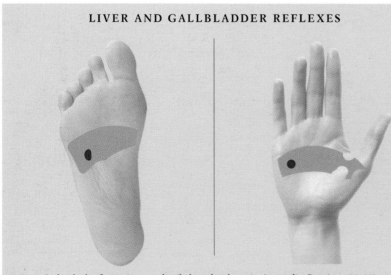

LIVER AND GALLBLADDER REFLEXES

Individual reflex points are detailed on the charts in Appendix One (pp.130–35).

HELPS BALANCE
CALCIUM LEVELS

ADRENAL GLAND REFLEX

Extra pressure on the adrenal gland reflex insures its powerful anti-inflammatory substances (see p. 51) are released.

PARATHYROID REFLEX

ADRENAL GLAND REFLEX

The thyroid and parathyroid hormones help to balance calcium levels; imbalances can be due to overactivity in the parathyroid glands (see p. 51), and any slight hiccup that occurs in this area can be the cause of calculus forming.

On the hand, if there is pain in the side areas of the abdomen, apply pressure on TB-3 (between the fourth and fifth knuckles).

APPLY
PRESSURE

TB-3 POINT

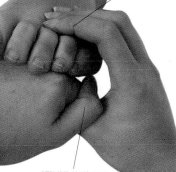

CAN HELP
PREVENT
GALLSTONES

STIMULATES BILE
PRODUCTION

**PARATHYROID REFLEX
ON UPPER SURFACE**

TB-3 POINT

On the leg, the Stomach meridian point ST-36 (four finger-widths below the knee, on the outside edge of the tibia bone) will relieve most abdominal pain, but do not use this point on young children.

Genitourinary Problems

BLADDER PROBLEMS *include infections such as cystitis and candida, which are often the result of stress, overwork, or overacidity. They may also be aggravated by cold weather. Disorders of the pelvic cavity include pelvic inflammatory disease, bloating, and menstrual disorders in women, and prostate problems in older men, of which urinary frequency, incontinence, or difficulty in passing urine are often the most distressing and painful symptoms.*

BLADDER PROBLEMS

Bladder problems are common, and include pain, discomfort, or bleeding when urinating. Many problems are due to infections that cause inflammation of the inner lining of the bladder. Urinary frequency may be due simply to stress, or to poor muscle tone in the pelvic floor, which is common in women around the time of childbirth. In cystitis, which is much more common in women, infection with *Escherichia coli* bacteria often occurs when the person is in a run-down condition. In men, benign enlargement of the prostate gland is frequently the cause (*see p. 123*).

KIDNEY REFLEX HELPS BALANCE URINARY ACIDITY

KIDNEY REFLEX

Areas to work

The main reflexes to work are the kidney and bladder reflexes, to balance the urinary acidity. Work the whole area, as infection can spread to other organs from the urinary tract, including the kidneys, the uterus, the vagina, and the small intestine. The bladder is a mass of blood and lymphatic vessels with a strong nerve supply. The bladder point is often red, raised, and puffy where there is a problem.

WORK THE BLADDER POINT TO AID BLADDER COMPLAINTS

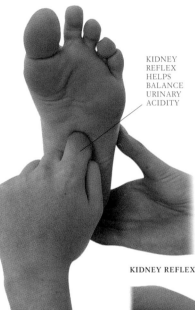

KIDNEY AND BLADDER REFLEXES

Individual reflex points are detailed on the charts in Appendix One (pp.130–35).

BLADDER REFLEX

LOWER SPINAL REFLEXES

Also work the lower spinal reflexes to help relax the pelvic nerves.

For inflammation, work the adrenal gland reflex. Extra pressure or rotation on this reflex point for a minute has a direct effect on the inflamed areas. Also work the spinal areas to stimulate the nerve supply to the pelvis.

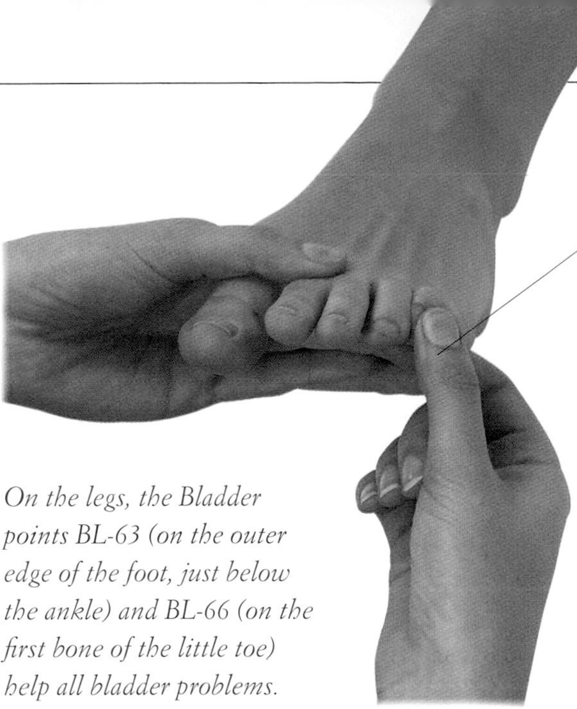

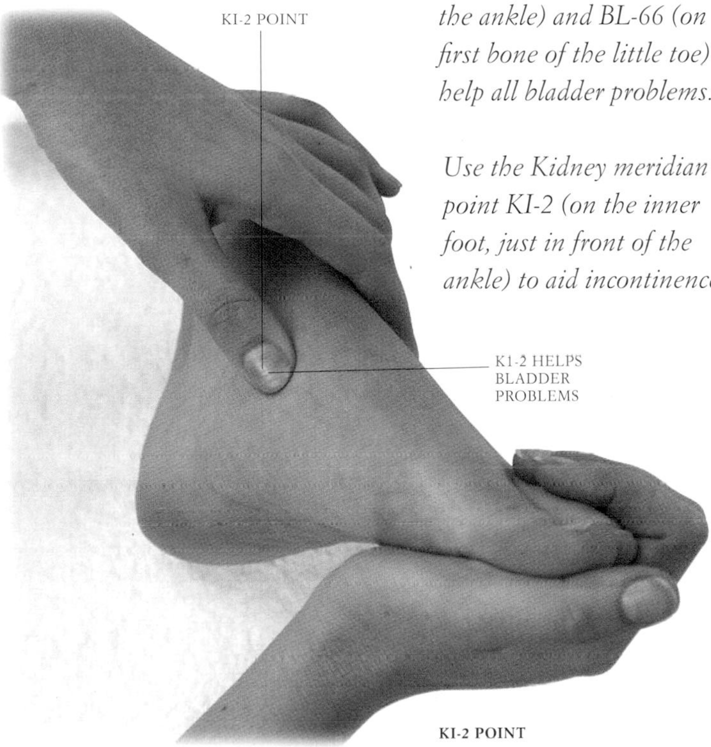

KI-2 POINT

K1-2 HELPS BLADDER PROBLEMS

KI-2 POINT

BL-66 POINT

On the legs, the Bladder points BL-63 (on the outer edge of the foot, just below the ankle) and BL-66 (on the first bone of the little toe) help all bladder problems.

Use the Kidney meridian point KI-2 (on the inner foot, just in front of the ankle) to aid incontinence.

BL-66 POINT

On the ear, use the pelvic point in the lower triangular fossa hollow and the kidney point on the back surface. The point in the angle of the upper concha is also used for infections of this tract.

LU-10

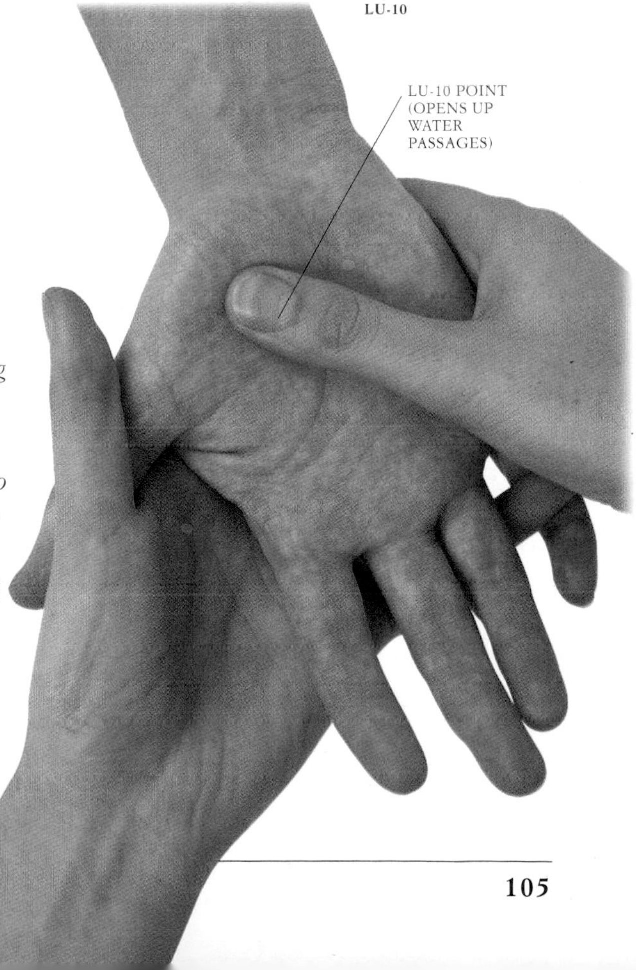

LU-10 POINT (OPENS UP WATER PASSAGES)

DIET

For cystitis, cranberry, blueberry, or boiled beetroot juice are helpful in preventing bacteria adhering to the bladder wall. Try to increase your general fluid intake, but remember that caffeinated food and drinks appear to irritate the urinary tissues.

On the hands, use the Lung point LU-10 (two thumb-widths below the wrist crease on the thumb pad) to open up the water passages and work the Large Intestine point LI-4 (found in the web between the thumb and forefinger), this has a calming and antispasmodic action.

CALCULI (STONES)

Kidney stones are the result of an imbalance in the renal tract. The kidneys are greatly affected by stress, which often reduces urine secretion. These stones are a mass of calcium phosphate crystals, calcium oxalate, and uric acid. They can be present for many years, but if stones pass into a duct, they can create a major problem, as the person suffers excruciating pain symptoms and surgery is then needed.

CAUTION

If there is severe pain, it is imperative to seek medical advice as soon as possible.

Areas to work

The thyroid and parathyroid hormones help to balance the calcium levels; overactivity in the parathyroid glands (see Endocrine system, pp. 50–51) can be the cause of calculus forming. If there is inflammation of the kidneys, work the thyroid/parathyroid point to balance calcium and phosphorus levels. The whole urinary system needs to be worked thoroughly, so it is advisable to seek help from a professional reflexologist.
Extra pressure on the adrenal gland

DIET

For kidney stones, calcium-forming foods should be limited. Avoid excess dairy products, such as cheese and milk, as you can obtain enough calcium from fresh green vegetables. Water intake should be increased, as low levels are often the cause of an imbalance; bottled water is better than tap water, which often contains higher levels of calcium. If you take part in any sport, try to avoid becoming too dehydrated, as this makes the urine much stronger. Aim to drink one to two quarts of water per day.

Apple and cranberry juice are beneficial drinks. Cranberry products, which are acidic in nature, help to keep the bacteria E. coli from adhering to the tissue of the bladder wall. Celery in any form aids elimination; it is an alkaline vegetable that is purported to be beneficial for any overacidity. To help alleviate candida avoid yeast and sugar-containing products. The correct diet will help enormously – cut out all refined carbohydrates and eat plenty of garlic, fresh green vegetables, and fruit.

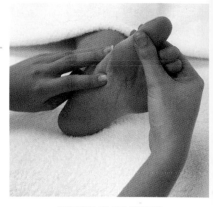

ADRENAL GLAND REFLEX

reflex insures its powerful anti-inflammatory substances (see pp. 50–51) are released; stimulation also aids the regular filtering and elimination process.

Working on the great toe or thumb will stimulate the pituitary/hypothalamus to encourage a balanced filtration within the network of blood vessels (capillaries) in the kidneys.

WORK ON THE
GREAT TOE FOR
PITUITARY REFLEX

PITUITARY REFLEX

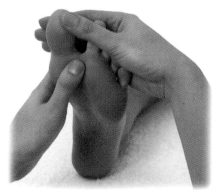

THYROID REFLEX

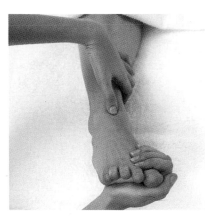

LOWER LYMPHATIC REFLEXES

> **CAUTION**
> Do not use SP-6 in
> pregnancy.

CANDIDA

Vaginal thrush is very common and is caused by the fungus *candida albicans* growing in the vagina.

Areas to work

For both males and females, work the lower lymphatic areas, the spleen, and intestines.

On the lower legs, the Spleen point SP-6 (four finger-widths above the inside ankle bone, just behind the tibia shin bone) helps with abdominal discomfort.

On the ears, use the point in the crease at the bottom of the concha hollow for its anti-inflammatory properties.

REPRODUCTIVE AND PELVIC PROBLEMS

General problems associated with the pelvic area include inflammation, bloating, and swelling (edema). Swelling is common in women before the menstrual period, and is often associated with food intolerance (especially wheat), but severe swelling can also be a symptom of a developing kidney disorder and should always be investigated medically.

Areas to work

Work the kidney reflex to remove excess fluid. For inflammation, work the adrenal reflex to stimulate its anti-inflammatory compounds.

On the lower legs, use the Spleen points SP-5 (in the depression in front of the inner ankle) for abdominal swelling, SP-6 (four finger-widths above bottom of the tibia shin bone, on the hind edge), and SP-9 (in the depression below the head of the tibia) for general pelvic disorders.

SP-6 POINT

RELIEVES
ABDOMINAL
DISCOMFORT

SP-6 POINT

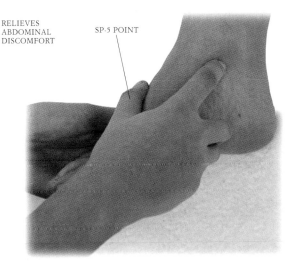

SP-5 POINT

SP-5 POINT

Circulatory Problems

HYPERTENSION IS ELEVATED ARTERIAL PRESSURE. *Hypotension is an abnormally low pressure of arterial blood. There may be problems with the heart itself, including degeneration of heart muscle with age or after infection (e.g., rheumatic fever), hardening (arteriosclerosis) or swelling and distortion (aneurysm) of the heart arteries, angina, and irregular beating (cardiac arrhythmia). There seems to be no one cause that increases the risk of a heart disorder; the many contributing factors include genetic predisposition, smoking, diet, and lack of exercise. Medical intervention may be needed to avoid more serious complications developing, but reflexology can also have a beneficial effect on the circulation.*

CARDIAC PROBLEMS

Coronary heart disease is one of the leading causes of premature death in the developed countries. It is caused by the build-up of fatty deposits in the arteries that supply the heart muscle with blood. Factors that contribute to the disease include a diet rich in saturated fats, high cholesterol levels, stress, lack of exercise, smoking, genetic make-up, and being overweight.

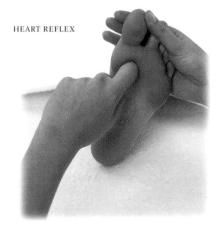

HEART REFLEX

Areas to work

Work the great toe to stimulate the circulation and the whole cardiac cycle. Work on the liver area on the sole of the foot or the palm of the hand to stimulate the release of bile salts, which normalize cholesterol levels. These also balance levels of different chemicals that come from the kidneys and adrenals and raise blood pressure. For problems with the heart itself, work the heart reflex.

CIRCULATORY REFLEXES

Individual reflex points are detailed on the charts in Appendix One (pp.130–35).

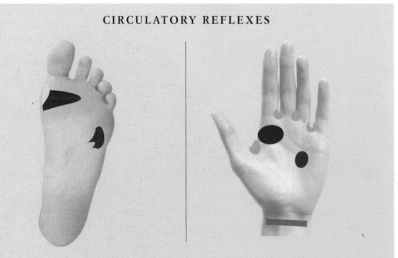

LIVER REFLEX

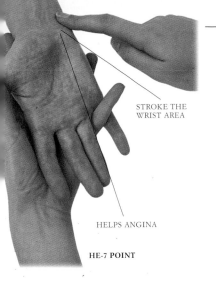

STROKE THE
WRIST AREA

HELPS ANGINA

HE-7 POINT

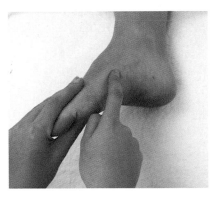

SP-4 POINT

DIET

Garlic is recommended for high blood pressure. Fish oils counteract cardiac arrhythmia, and they also thin the blood, reducing the risk of blood clotting. Other oils (e.g., vegetable oils) increase the "stickiness" of the blood and its tendency to clot.

To help angina and any increase in the heart rate above normal, stroke the wrist area, below the little finger, over the creases; then apply pressure on the inner forearm, between the tendons, a palm's width up the arm. The following acupoints also help:
(i) The Lung point LU-9 (on the thumb side of the wrist crease) benefits the blood vessels.
(ii) The Pericardium point PE-4 (one hand's-width above the wrist on the inner forearm) will regulate and strengthen the heartbeat; PE-9 (on the tip of the middle finger) is used to treat aneurysm.
(iii) The Heart meridian should be worked from HE-9 (on the inside tip of the little finger) to HE-4 (just above the wrist); HE-9 is indicated for palpitations.
(iv) On the wrist, the Shenmen point (HE-7, on the little-finger side of the wrist crease) is used for calming.

On the sole of the foot, the first Kidney point (KI-1, in the crease in the middle of the ball of the foot) is a vital point for hypertension. It is also very calming. The Spleen point SP-4 (at the proximal end of the first metatarsal bone) aids the spleen, which, according to T.C.M. theory, is the organ most closely associated with the blood; SP-4 also specifically alleviates cardiac inflammation.

On the ear, a point in the upper triangular fossa hollow will lower blood pressure. The point in the center of the upper concha is used for any circulatory disorder. The point in the center of the ear (on both front and back surfaces) will contact the vagus nerve (see p. 63) directly; this has the effect of slowing the heartbeat.

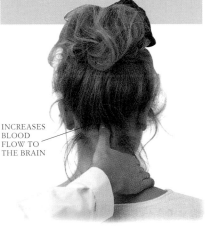

INCREASES
BLOOD
FLOW TO
THE BRAIN

GV-16 POINT

On the back of the head, either side of the above point are the Fengchi points (GB-20). These are potent in lowering blood pressure and neck and head related problems.

PE-4 POINT

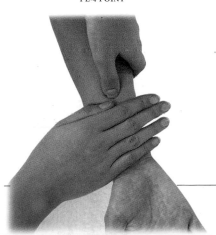

TRIANGULAR
FOSSA POINT
IS GOOD FOR
CIRCULATORY
PROBLEMS

**TRIANGULAR
FOSSA POINT**

Allergies, Eczema, and Skin Problems

THE BODY CAN REACT BADLY *to a variety of different substances in the environment, including specific foods, pollen or grasses, dust, and chemicals. Allergies can cause many physical reactions, creating inflammation, causing bloating, or irritating mucous membranes in the eyes, ears, or nose (as in allergic rhinitis). The last of these effects will result in excessive production of large amounts of mucus (which is produced as a protective measure); this, in turn, will cause clogging of various internal tracts. Diarrhea is also a symptom that can indicate a variety of allergic problems.*

ECZEMA AND OTHER SKIN PROBLEMS

It is not possible to describe all skin problems and the object is not to diagnose any of these disorders, but instead to show how a relaxed state can improve even the most chronic skin problems. For acute eczema (where the skin is covered in tiny blisters with extreme redness, or crusting), the hands can usually be worked successfully. This will soon stimulate the production of new skin. A water spray can also be used on all areas of the feet to stimulate the reflexes. Care must be taken, however, as too much pressure can cause discomfort and may cause the skin to split even more.

Sources of stress should also be considered, as most people do not realize that the skin disorder is often the outcome of allergies or extreme stress and anxiety that is present in their everyday lives. Refer also to Stress (*see pp. 86–87*) and Children's Health ailments for acne (*see p. 116*).

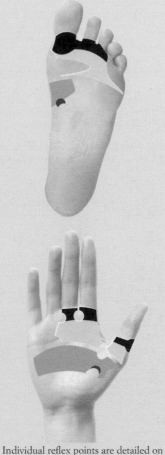

ALLERGY REFLEXES

Individual reflex points are detailed on the charts in Appendix One (pp.130–35).

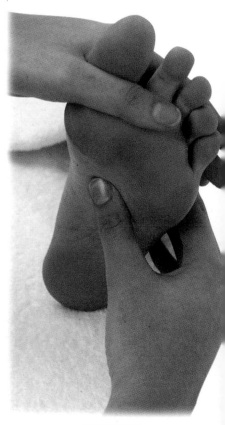

Areas to work
Work the left lobe of the liver. According to T.C.M., this lobe has a regulating function.

LIVER REFLEX

WORK THE
LUNG REFLEX

LUNG REFLEX

Start by working the lung reflex area on either hands or feet. On the hands, this is on the pads of the palm below the fingers; on the feet, it is on the ball of the foot.

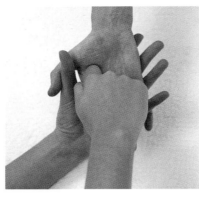

ADRENAL GLAND REFLEX

Also work any of the adrenal points. The adrenal gland reflex can be found in the hand on the base of the web between the thumb and index finger on the palmar surface only. On the feet, it lays in the upper arch on the inner edge. Work either of these reflexes for a few minutes.

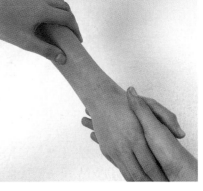

TB-6 POINT

On the arm, a point on the Triple Burner meridian (TB-6, in the middle of the back of the forearm, four thumb-widths up from the wrist crease) is ideal for all skin eruptions, including eczema.

POINT ON
OUTER TIP OF
EAR ALLEVIATES
INFLAMMATION

ADRENAL GLAND POINT

POINT ON
FRONTAL
CARTILAGE
CALMS
PERSISTENT
ITCHING

WIND STREAM POINT

*On the ear are two useful points:
(i) On the outer tip of the ear, the Wind Stream point helps any allergy and skin irritation.
(ii) A point on the frontal cartilage projection stimulates production of anti-inflammatory substances by the adrenal glands, calming the most persistent itching.*

GENERAL ALLERGIES

Allergies are extremely common. They occur when the body's immune system is hypersensitive to harmless substances known as allergens. Common allergens include pollen, house-dust mites, animals, and certain foods (for example, nuts or shellfish). Allergic symptoms include wheezing, headaches, a runny nose, itchy eyes, and rashes (*see p. 31*).

Areas to work

For all kinds of allergies, the adrenal glands need to be stimulated, because it is here that the natural anti-inflammatory substance cortisone is produced. The adrenal gland reflex can be found in the hand, on the base of the web between the thumb and index finger on the palmar surface only. On the feet, it lays in the upper arch on the inner edge. Work either of these reflexes for a few minutes.

DIET

It is best to restrict all mucus-forming foods. Eat lots of wholefoods and vegetables, and very little fish or meat. Sugar should be excluded from the diet, as this may encourage skin fungal growth. Stimulants such as coffee, tea, and alcohol should be limited, but at least two quarts of water should be drunk daily. Dandelion tea is extremely beneficial as it cleanses the liver, which is important for all high toxicity conditions, including eczema and urticaria. If there are high mucus levels, eating papaya fruit will help break it down.

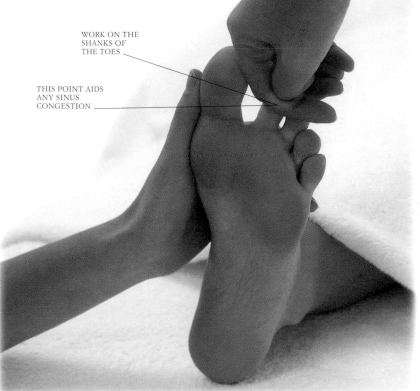

WORK ON THE SHANKS OF THE TOES

THIS POINT AIDS ANY SINUS CONGESTION

For symptoms in the head, work the shanks of the toes and the fingers; this area corresponds to the sinus, ear, and eye regions. The main aim is to correct excessive mucus production, reducing the swelling in the mucous membranes. Working this area also has a sedative action on the brain, which helps to settle a ticklish cough.

REDUCES SWELLING AND MUCUS PRODUCTION

CAUTION

LI-4 is a point with a powerful action and must not be used during pregnancy, as it is used to promote delivery during labor.

WORK THE SHANKS OF THE FINGERS

REFLEX FOR HEAD–RELATED AREAS

STIMULATE
THE LU-10
POINT TO
ALLEVIATE
ASTHMA

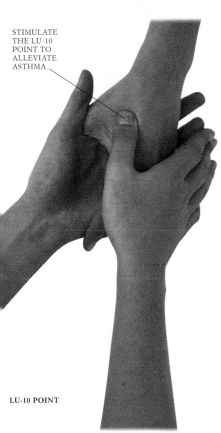

LU-10 POINT

On the ear, a point on the cartilage projection above the lobe will alleviate inflammation. The Wind Stream point (in the scaphoid fossa) is specific for allergies; the Ear Shenmen (in the triangular fossa hollow) is another point to use (see also p.64). The adrenal reflex point is found on the frontal cartilage projection of the ear.

HELPS ALLERGIC
DISORDERS

On the face, a point on the Large Intestine meridian (LI-20, either side of the nostrils) is useful for allergic rhinitis (nasal inflammation).

WIND STREAM

This is LU-10 which helps to clear mucus in the throat and aid asthma.

On the hand, two acupoints give further relief from pain:
(i) A point on the Large Intestine meridian LI-4 (on the back of the hand in the web between the thumb and index finger, see p. 91) gives almost instant relief, helping to prevent the excessive swelling of the many blood vessels involved, often reducing redness as this point. It also aids ears and eyes and alleviates hayfever.
(ii) For allergic skin reactions, use a point on the Triple Burner meridian (TB-6, four finger-widths above the wrist on the back of the forearm).

LI-20 POINT

THIS POINT
HELPS NASAL
INFLAMMATION

LI-20 POINT

113

Reflexology for Particular Groups

The therapeutic touch of reflexology can help with all kinds of specific problems, from childhood teething to adolescent acne, from genitourinary conditions in both men and women, to the aches and pains that are felt in advancing years.

Many specific problems in both the young and elderly are caused by nutritional deficiencies. Food allergies in the young have become alarmingly common, and although this may in part be due to incorrect eating, we now know that many additives and colorings can affect children's behavior. The usual response is hyperactivity, but in more severe cases children can experience learning difficulties and emotional instability that stay with them throughout their lives. Allergens have mutated and become quite diverse, causing allergies and food intolerances that can lead to unpleasant, if transient, problems, such as diarrhea and constipation, or severe and abnormal responses, such as anaphylactic shock (a severe reaction to injected foreign material) and chronic food poisoning.

Most of us treat ourselves with scant respect and only begin to show our bodies a little more consideration when we become ill or a problem arises. Yet if we look at ourselves, we will find that our bodies are miracles that should be treated with reverence and care. If we have low self-esteem or self-image, then, regardless of age, we will be more prone to disease. Ulcers or high blood pressure are either hereditary conditions or are a consequence of our lifestyle; we do not catch them like a common cold. However, even a common cold is more likely to develop if we are run down and suffering from fatigue, anxiety, or stress.

Many health hazards threaten our daily life, causing our immune systems to become depleted. Reflexology helps us to resist these invisible and implacable invaders by boosting our immune systems, enhancing heart circulation and cardiovascular performance, and improving oxygen consumption so that organs can function at an optimal level. Indeed, if reflexology were practiced from youth through to old age, it would act as a natural preventative to disease, giving us a much better quality of life and an innate sense of true well-being.

REFLEXOLOGY PRACTITIONER

REFLEXOLOGY HELPS PEOPLE OF ALL AGE GROUPS

TREATMENT CAN HELP MANY DIFFERENT PROBLEMS

LEFT *Disorders associated with the menstrual cycle can be alleviated with reflexology treatment.*

Children's Health

GENTLE TREATMENT *on all areas of the foot or hand will aid and strengthen the child's immune system, giving protection from coughs and colds and many minor but irritating problems. A general workout will often lower a high temperature and, as it is very calming, will alleviate night-time disturbances, fretfulness, and other emotional problems. Observe how the tiniest babies involuntarily respond to touch – their little fingers or toes will curl around your fingers as you apply gentle pressure – working on their hands or feet can create a reassuring sense of bonding.*

BABIES AND INFANTS

Gentle stretching of fingers and toes will stimulate all head-related areas. Working on the base of the big toe will aid digestion and calm any anxieties in the most distressed child. This gentle stretching and rotation of each finger and toe will contact all the 10 zones and 12 meridians. Gently working on the hands or feet with a caressing, feather-like touch will have a calming action on the whole body, and if a child is fretful or has a slight temperature, this exercise should reduce it quite quickly.

Infantile colic is a distressing problem, both for the baby and for the new parents, as they often feel helpless because they cannot relieve the discomfort of the crying infant; this is often caused by wind while feeding. Sitting for a few minutes prior to feeding and stroking the hands and feet can settle the most restless child and relieve the colic.

BELOW *Most childhood illnesses will respond to the therapeutic touch of reflexology.*

DIET

It is important to establish a good diet, as food can often cause problems throughout the early years. For instance, eating processed foods, or foods that are high in hidden sugars, often leads to a clogged intestinal state. Some foods, such as milk, are causative factors in respiratory and sinus problems. Diet should include plenty of soluble fiber, including fruit. Minimize processed foods, but increase fluid intake considerably to at least six glasses of water throughout the day. To combat common viral infections, eating foods that are high in vitamin C, which therefore have an antiviral effect, should be encouraged.

CAUTION

Make sure that you apply only gentle pressure; do not press as hard as you would on an adult patient.

SCHOOL-AGE CHILDREN

When children are a little older, all their common illnesses can be treated with a gentle general treatment, that will often lower high temperatures and ease any fretfulness. Work the reflex area of the problem and also stimulate the skeletal area, as this will in turn stimulate the lymphatic circulation (*see pp. 60–61*). It is crucial also that the thyroid gland functions well, as the hormones it produces are an essential part of normal mental and physical development, and imbalances can affect the hair, skin, and nails.

Regular reflexology aids the child's mental development, also, as it gives the added assurance of the continued physical contact. Children frequently go through particularly traumatic emotions during their first school years, and this may cause other problems. Constipation, for instance, is a common distressing problem. This can lead to other distressing symptoms such as soiling, or pain due to hard, compressed stools. Reflexology can help by relieving the stress of the situation.

Work the hands daily to help most of the irritating daily problems. When you are washing the child's ears, use a washcloth, giving them a good rub to stimulate the ear reflex points (*see pp. 64–65*).

PUBERTY

Puberty and the teenage years can bring more problems, as hormone levels are changing dramatically and some children also find the change from child to adult quite distressing. During this period, young adults may feel that their parents do not understand them, and this is when contact can be lost, as kissing and hugging are looked upon as babyish behavior. Reflexology can restore this physical contact.

Acne is a common problem during puberty, and this can create its own stresses. Even if continual hygiene is observed, troublesome skin can still appear. Reflexology helps to calm the sebaceous glands and the circulating hormones. Stimulation to the pituitary, thyroid, and the adrenal gland reflexes helps to balance these hormones, mainly testosterone in males and the ovarian hormones in females.

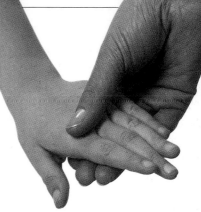

ABOVE *Children love to be touched on their hands or feet.*

Areas to work

Work the reflex area of the problem. Working over the diaphragm reflex relaxes the breathing during infections; also work the cervical reflex at the side of the great toe or the hand just below the nail bed to relax the neck down to the diaphragm.
Stimulation to the back of the ear will trigger the vagus nerve (see p. 63) into action; this nerve supplies the respiratory processes with nervous stimulation, and working this area will also help to relax the breathing.

CAUTION

It cannot be stressed enough that any undue pain or abnormal disturbance in your child should be referred to your local medical practitioner. For any disorder of young children, it is imperative to seek medical advice before giving any treatment, if in doubt about the cause of the complaint.

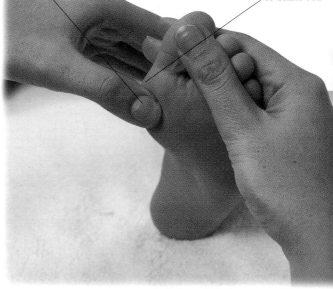

DIAPHRAGM REFLEX

WORK AT SIDE OF GREAT TOE

DIAPHRAGM REFLEX

For a temperature, the hypothalamus/pituitary point should be worked on the great toe; this reflex controls the autonomic functions and the regulation of body temperature, and gentle rotation on this point will help to lower a raised temperature.

Working on the foot on the second Spleen meridian point SP-2 (almost at the base of the great toe) will help any agitation.

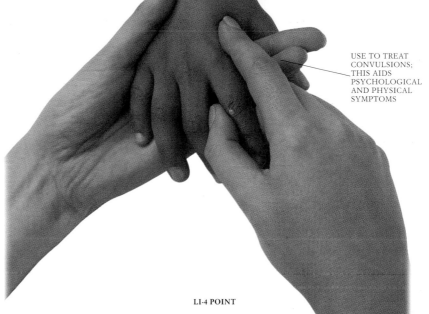

USE TO TREAT CONVULSIONS; THIS AIDS PSYCHOLOGICAL AND PHYSICAL SYMPTOMS

LI-4 POINT

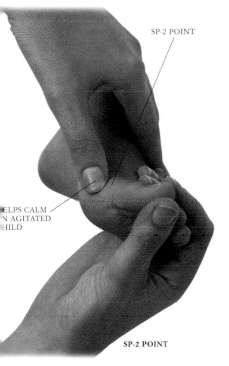

SP-2 POINT

ELPS CALM
N AGITATED
HILD

SP-2 POINT

Working the thymus reflex will help the whole immune response; do gentle rotation from the neck reflex down to the diaphragm line on both hands and feet. As children get older, this area can be worked several times daily whenever there are any infections present. Working the thymus area also aids any agitation in young children. Remember that you should barely caress the surface in tiny babies.

Barely stroke the thyroid reflex, as it generally needs to be soothed. There is a complex connection between the thyroid gland, the nervous system, and the rate of metabolic processes (see pp. 50–51), and thyroid imbalances can also affect the condition of the hair, skin, and nails.

For convulsions, the Large Intestine point LI-4 on the hand (in the web between the thumb and index finger), and, on the foot, the Liver points LIV-1 to LIV-2, at the base of the web between the great and second toe, (see p. 118), and LIV-3 (at the lowest point between the two bones), a calming point, may be used. The first Kidney point, KI-1 (found in the depression behind the ball of the foot, or on the little toe as the meridian also arises there) is a good balancing point to use for any feelings of fretfulness.

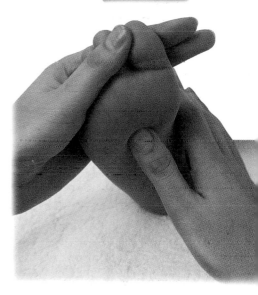

KI-1 POINT

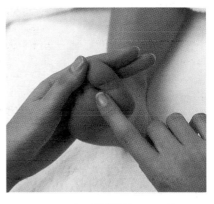

LINEITING: NEW POINT FOR CONVULSIONS

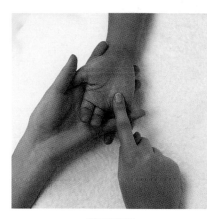

HE-8 POINT

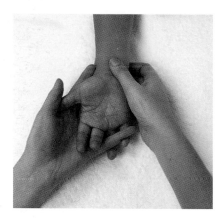

PE-6 POINT

TEETHING PROBLEMS
For troublesome teething problems, work down the second toe to contact the Stomach meridian points ST-44 (on the top of the foot in the web between the second and third toes),

TROUBLED SLEEP
For bad dreams or other night-time disturbances, work on the palm of the hand to stimulate the Heart meridian point HE-8 (in line with the base of the thumb web below the fourth and little finger)

DIGESTIVE DISORDERS
Minor digestive disorders can be helped by working the Pericardium point PE-6 (two thumb-widths up from the palm side of the wrist crease on the inner forearm); this balances the liver and calms tummy problems.

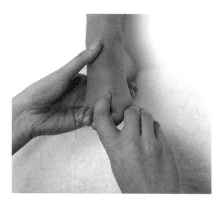

ST-44 POINT

ST-45 (lateral side of the second toe base of nail bed) is also good for teething.

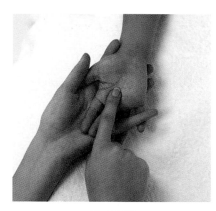

PE-8 POINT

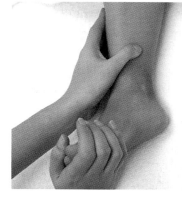

SP-6 POINT

The Pericardium point PE-8 (at the same level as HE-8, below the middle or big finger) will also help to guard against nightmares. Both are good calming points and will also help if there is a slight temperature.

ABDOMINAL PAIN
For older children, to relieve abdominal pain the Spleen meridian point SP-6 (four finger-widths above the inner ankle bone) can be worked.

LIV-2 FOR
INSOMNIA,
TOOTHACHE

LIV-1 FOR
CONSTIPATION

LIV-1 AND LIV-2 POINTS

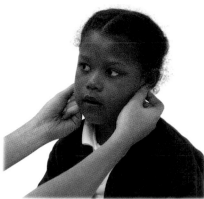

TOOTH REFLEX

MEDIAL EDGE

On the medial edge of the ear is a another good point for teeth; gently apply pressure on this point for general discomfort in the facial area. Perhaps this is why young children pull their ears when they are teething.

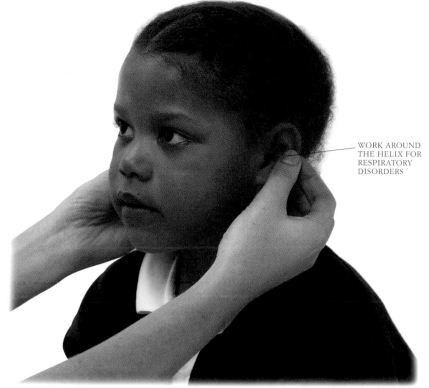

WORK AROUND THE HELIX FOR RESPIRATORY DISORDERS

RESPIRATORY REFLEX

RESPIRATORY DISORDERS

For respiratory disorders, work all around the helix (the outer, curved, fleshy ridge of the ear); this also helps tonsillitis and fever. On the foot, the Stomach meridian point ST-45 (see p.118) aids tonsillitis.

Refer also to the sections on Respiratory Problems (see pp. 94–97), Bladder Problems (see p. 104), and Ear Problems (see p. 92).

SKIN PROBLEMS

For skin eruptions, apply gentle pressure on the hands to a point on the Triple Burner meridian TB-6 (four finger-widths above the wrist on the back of the forearm).

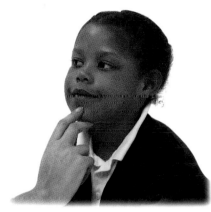

REFLEX FOR CONSTIPATION

CONSTIPATION

If a child is constipated, apply gentle pressure at the base of the lower lip in the upper cleft of the chin. Also rotate on LIV-1.

TB-6 POINT

TB-6 POINT USED TO TREAT SKIN ERUPTIONS

Female Problems

PROBLEMS THAT ARE SPECIFIC TO WOMEN *include the menstrual disorders from which very many women suffer at some time in their lives. They also suffer unnecessarily during pregnancy. Breast problems, such as general discomfort, swelling, or lumpiness, also come and go with the menstrual cycle. All of these problems can be alleviated with reflexology.*

BREAST PROBLEMS

Most breast problems are caused by hormonal imbalances. Small lumps may be due to cystic mastitis. However, all such problems should be investigated by a medical practitioner to eliminate any possible malignancy. The following treatments can be used to help alleviate general breast discomfort:

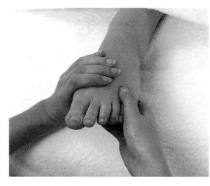

GB-42 POINT

Areas to work

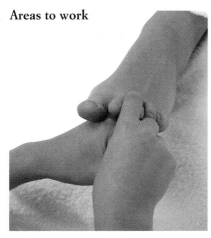

BREAST REFLEX

On the legs, for mastitis and the axillary areas, use a point on the Gallbladder meridian (GB-42, on the top of the foot in the furrow between the fourth and fifth toes).

On the ears, use the endocrine point (located in the front crease of the lower concha).

ENDOCRINE REFLEX

Work the axillary and breast area between the second and third toes, and the upper lymphatics area.

On the hands, the Large Intestine point LI-4 (in the web between the thumb and first finger) will help the axillary area.

MENSTRUAL PROBLEMS

These include amenorrhea (scanty or absent periods), dysmenorrhea (painful periods), premenstrual syndrome (P.M.S.), and pelvic inflammatory disease. There may also be distressing symptoms associated with the menopause (hot flashes, vaginal dryness, mood changes). Most such problems are due to imbalances in hormonal levels. Vasodilation (dilation of blood vessels), congestion, and salt water imbalances in the tissues also play a part. Reflexology can give deep muscle relaxation, quick pain relief, and in the longer term can help to normalize hormonal levels. Exercise and a healthy diet are also important.

CAUTION

Avoid point SP-6 during pregnancy.

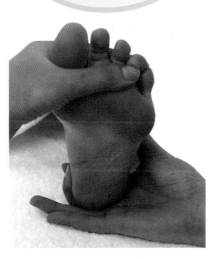

UTERUS REFLEX

DIET

A high fat diet increases estrogen levels, as estrogen is partly derived from fat and cholesterol. A monounsaturated fat, such as olive oil, is a good choice if you need to increase your levels. Evening primrose or starflower oil is helpful for P.M.S., as is a high carbohydrate diet. Some plant foods, such as soybean products and linseed, contain estrogen-like substances and can alleviate menopausal symptoms. Menopausal women need to insure that their diet contains sufficient calcium, magnesium, and boron. Green vegetables such as broccoli and green beans contain calcium, and nuts contain magnesium and boron, as does fruit such as apples.

Areas to work

Work all the reproductive areas and the endocrine reflex. For any inflammation, also work the adrenal reflex. Work the kidney reflex to remove any excess fluid and swelling.

On the hands, the Large Intestine point LI-4 (in the web between the thumb and forefinger) alleviates spasm in the uterus.

On the legs, the Spleen meridian point SP-1 calms spasm in the uterus. SP- 6, and 9 (running up the inside of the foot and leg) help to normalize menstruation.

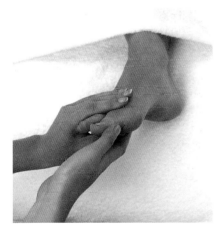

SP-1 POINT

FALLOPIAN AND GROIN REFLEX

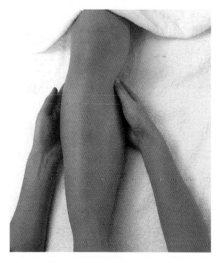

SP-9 POINT

PREGNANCY AND LABOR

Reflexology employed throughout pregnancy helps to insure a healthy, trouble-free time, although regular health checks should be continued. Regular therapy relieves the minor aches and pains caused by the many changes that the body undergoes at this time. It can aid morning sickness, constipation, back pain, and emotional upsets, which may cause headaches or anxiety. Also, it often increases energy levels. High blood pressure can also frequently be avoided. Reflexology can, in addition, help those who wish to give birth by "natural" methods, as it assists relaxation and dilatation of the uterine muscular wall. People who use reflexology throughout their pregnancies often seem less likely to suffer tears, as the treatment relaxes the perineal muscles.

As far back as 1917, Dr. Fitzgerald advocated applying pressure for painless childbirth. He stated that zonal pressure was a boon to womankind, and devised grips and clamps for the hands and feet, to apply the required pressure. He also spoke of applying pressure over the the great toe (the acupoint SP-1, which relieves spasms of the uterus), and advocated the firm stroking of the back of the hand to assist the afterbirth and relieve morning sickness.

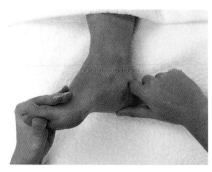

SPINAL REFLEX

Areas to work

PREGNANCY

For low back pain and soreness, work the spinal areas and the musculature of the hip/pelvis (see also Musculoskeletal problems, p. 80–81).

On the arms, the Lung meridian point LU-8 (just above the wrist crease, on the thumb side) and the Pericardium point PE-6 (two thumb-widths above the wrist crease in the middle of the inner forearm) help to subdue vomiting and morning sickness.

> **CAUTION**
> Never use points SP-6, or BL-60 during pregnancy at all, or LI-4 up to week 38 as they may induce premature labor and miscarriage.

> **CAUTION**
> The Large Intestine point LI-4 can safely be used from week 38 onward.

LABOR

On the hands, the Large Intestine point LI-4 (in the web of the thumb and first finger) relieves spasms of the uterus.

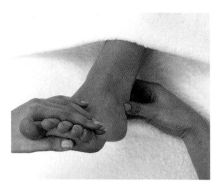

BL-60 POINT

On the legs, the Bladder meridian point BL-60 (around the outside ankle bone) will not only aid any back discomfort, but also promote delivery. The Spleen meridian point SP-6 (four finger-widths above the bottom of the tibia leg bone, on the rear edge) helps in the reduction of pain in the uterus, and also calms; work the area before and during contractions. For mastitis, use the Gallbladder point GB-42 (on the top of the foot in the furrow between the fourth and fifth bones).

On the ears, the points at the ear apex and on the lower cartilage projection are useful for mastitis.

On the shoulder, the Gallbladder point GB-21 (found in the depression on the shoulders) will aid in the final stages of labor, as well as in promoting release of the afterbirth.

STROKING BACK
OF HAND

Male Prostate Problems

SYMPTOMS OF PROSTATE DYSFUNCTION *include the increased frequency of urination, the slowing of flow, and the need to strain, or pain while passing urine, possibly a slight fever, abdominal discomfort, and leakage. Reflexology treatment is aimed at relieving spasm in the bladder muscles, relaxing the sphincter muscles, and improving nerve impulses to the area.*

Areas to work

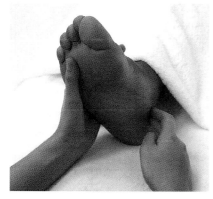

PROSTATE REFLEX

Work the prostate reflex, and other connected reflexes such as the bladder and rectum. The adrenal reflexes are also useful for inflammation.

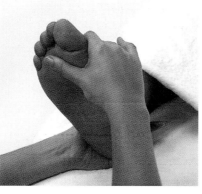

PROSTATE ROTATION

Prostate rotation relieves pain in the perineal area, aiding any prostate problems.

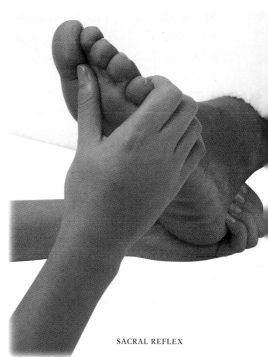

SACRAL REFLEX

The spinal reflexes, specifically the sacral area, should be worked to tone the sphincter muscles.

Working the rectum reflex induces stimulation from the sigmoid colon to the anal canal. This will aid defecation and help to eliminate any internal pressure on the prostate gland.

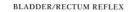

BLADDER/RECTUM REFLEX

123

The Elderly

IN AGING, THE INTERNAL ORGANS lose their elasticity and blood vessels tend to become thicker and more brittle, making them less able to function and causing the elderly to feel the cold more. This, in turn, may restrict the flow of blood to vital areas such as the heart and brain. The joints and ligaments also become stiff and less lubricated as we age, and many elderly people suffer from rheumatism and arthritis.

Areas to work

All areas of the hands and ears can be worked daily to promote general well-being. There are many gentle exercises of the hands and feet that can be done daily to retain flexibility (see p. 74–75).

Work the thyroid/parathyroid reflexes for arthritis and bone disorders. Stimulation to the adrenal reflexes aids in any inflammation.

In China, many centenarians advocate diet, breathing exercises, and the cultivation of inner peace and tranquility. Today, Tai Chi and qigong, two of these ancient exercise systems, are available for practice in the West, and are becoming increasingly popular. They are gentle exercises, suitable for all ages, and are widely considered to prolong life and help prevent and cure diseases that are age-related.

Reflexology also gives the body system a workout, endows a feeling of relaxation, and promotes a sense of well-being. Many long-standing problems such as arthritis or rheumatism can be relieved to some extent. It helps to strengthen the body's resistance to illness. Also, the joints feel more flexible, the nerve pathways are stimulated and thus the blood circulation is increased. (*See Musculoskeletal problems, pp. 80–81*)

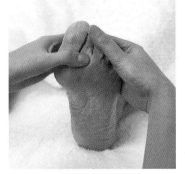

**THYROID/PARATHYROID
REFLEXES**

HELPS
INFLAMMATION

**UPPER AND LOWER
SURFACES**

RIGHT *Age-related diseases, such as rheumatism and osteoporosis, will benefit from regular reflexology treatment.*

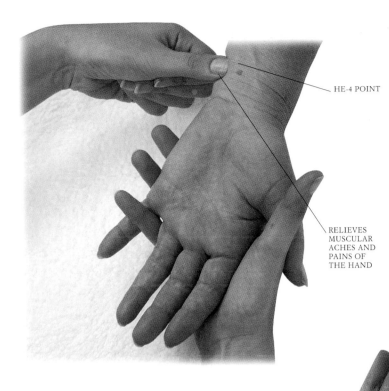

HE-4 POINT

RELIEVES MUSCULAR ACHES AND PAINS OF THE HAND

On the hands, use the Heart meridian point HE-4 (two finger-widths above the wrist crease on the elbow side) for muscular aches and pains between the wrist and elbow. The Triple Burner points TB-1 (at the base of the nail bed of the ring finger, outside edge) and TB-5 (two thumb-widths above the wrist crease) help arthritis of the upper trunk and shoulder.

HE-4 POINT

TB-5 POINT

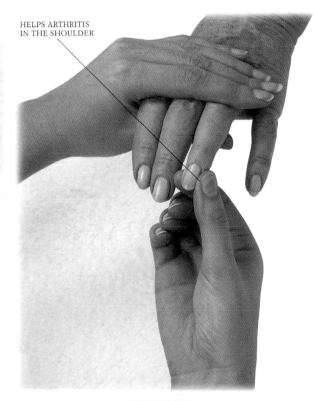

HELPS ARTHRITIS IN THE SHOULDER

TB-1 POINT (RING FINGER)

DIET

With age, the production of digestive enzymes tends to fall, so restraint in the diet is prudent; natural, easily digested foods such as fish and wholegrain cereals, which provide roughage, are beneficial. Foods high in calcium (e.g., leafy green vegetables, broccoli), nuts, fruits, and fatty fish, help prevent osteoporosis, while excess salt and coffee can rob your bones of calcium.

Visiting a Reflexologist

ALTHOUGH MANY CONDITIONS WILL IMPROVE *from self-help reflexology, there will be occasions when it would be advisable to visit a professional for treatment. This section describes what you can expect from such a visit, and answers some of the questions you may have.*

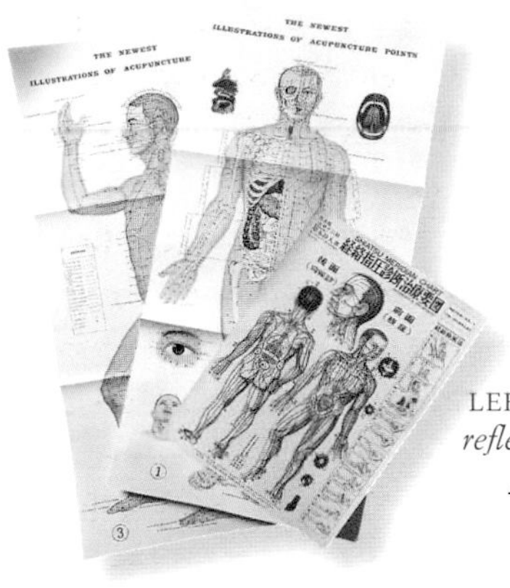

LEFT *Visit a professional reflexologist for treatment from time to time.*

CHOOSING A PRACTITIONER

A question people frequently ask is: "How do I find a registered practitioner?" Your national Medical Association will give the following recommendations:

Check to see whether the practitioner is with one of the leading organizations (*see p. 141*). If the practitioner belongs to an association, check to see whether this is independent from the training school, and for any letters after the person's name, as some training schools issue their own certificates that are not generally recognized.

Representative organizations should have a code of conduct for practice, someone who can deal with any complaints, and a

HOW MUCH DOES IT COST?

Another common question is: "How much should I pay for a treatment session?" Prices vary depending on whether you attend a practitioner's home or clinic. In health clubs or beauty salons the price can double to cover the costs of extra overheads.

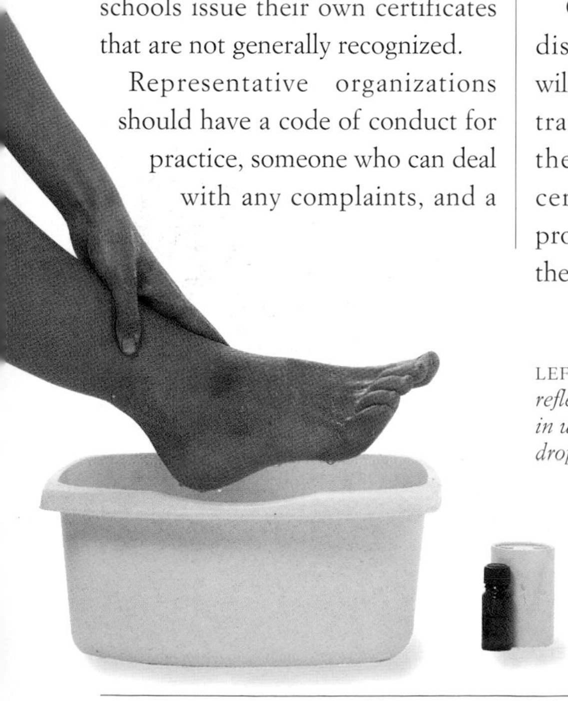

disciplinary procedure.

Good practitioners should display their certificates and be willing to tell you the depth of their training. They should also display their insurance and first aid certificates and those of any professional organizations to which they may belong.

LEFT *Before visiting a reflexologist, bathe your feet in warm water with a few drops of tea tree oil.*

PREPARATION FOR VISITING A THERAPIST

Prior to visiting a reflexologist, it is advisable to check your own feet to insure that the practitioner can work on all areas. Examine the area between each of the toes; broken skin could harbor a fungal infection. To discourage this, bathe your feet in warm water with three drops of antifungal tea tree oil. After washing, carefully dry between the toes and add a little foot powder. Shoes can exacerbate the problem, especially sneakers, which create a moist environment. Wearing shoes made of a natural material will allow the feet to breathe. Never share your towels, and change your socks or stockings daily as additional precautionary measures.

Do not be embarrassed if your feet tend to sweat profusely. Hyperhidrosis (excessive sweating) of the feet and hands is often stress-related and frequently occurs when the sympathetic nervous system (*see pp. 20–21*) is overactive. It is one of the clinical signs that a practitioner looks out for.

THE EXAMINATION

There are certain things you can expect a reflexologist to ask you. First, the practitioner will take a detailed case history, asking both general questions about your lifestyle – diet, smoking, tea, coffee, and alcohol consumption, exercise, and sleep patterns – and questions about your general health, including any allergies, emotional state, stress levels, blood pressure, injuries, or operations. If you have a particular complaint you wish to have treated, the practitioner will need to assess whether this is acute or chronic, or whether it is inherited.

Your feet and hands will then be examined closely; any marks or imperfections on them may indicate an imbalance within that area. Tender spots can be a signal of a problem in the functioning of the corresponding organ. If you have any pain, the practitioner will ask about its nature, location, and severity, and will also move the joints of your hands and feet to see their degree of movement.

It should be noted, however, that the reflexology analysis is not a conclusive medical diagnosis, but rather gives the practitioner an overall guideline to your health and mobility, and indications of specific areas to treat.

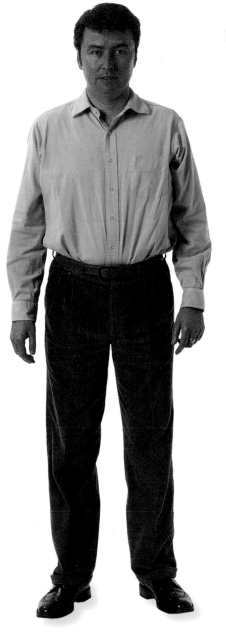

A CASE HISTORY

A heavy, stressful workload had left Kevin suffering from bouts of depression and sleepless nights. He constantly felt drained and found that he could not summon up any enthusiasm for life. The conventional medication prescribed by his physician was having very little positive effect – sleeping pills insured a good night's sleep but did not tackle his anxiety and depression.

He decided to consult a trained reflexologist in order to take a holistic approach to his imbalance.

Before beginning the treatment, the reflexologist took a detailed case history and discussed his lifestyle including his diet, exercise regime, emotional state, stress levels, and past injuries or operations.

After four weekly treatments, pinpointing certain areas that would induce relaxation and feelings of calm, Kevin reported that he was gradually beginning to feel more relaxed and positive about life. Kevin now visits his reflexologist on a monthly basis.

LEFT *Kevin's feelings of depression gradually began to lift after four weekly reflexology sessions.*

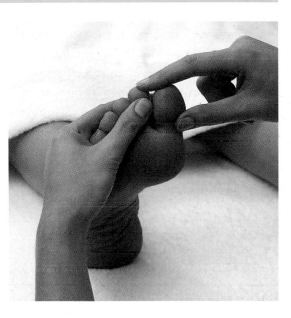

RIGHT *A reflexologist will examine your feet and hands closely for any imperfections or imbalances.*

THE TREATMENT

Usually the first reflexology session takes over an hour. This will allow time for the practitioner to ask you questions about your lifestyle and general health. Subsequent sessions may last from 30 to 50 minutes, according to the practitioner. If you need to rest after the treatment, you should be able to sit in another room, or you could get someone else to drive you to the session so that you can relax afterward.

RIGHT *A reflexology session will last from 30 to 50 minutes, according to the needs of the patient.*

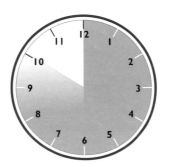

Most reflexologists work on the feet. However, they should also be able to utilize the hands or ears if, for some reason, it is difficult to work on the feet. They will also work on these areas as back-up areas. Specific "cross-reflexes" may also be employed when there is difficulty applying pressure to the area indicated; these are points in other areas of the body that are related to the primary areas, either by an anatomical or physiological connection.

Most people are amazed that the treatment does not feel ticklish and that they can immediately relax. Sometimes there is a feeling of warmth in the area being worked on, or nerve sensations (e.g., a little electric-type shock up the limb). If a tender spot is discovered, the reflexologist may work this several times during the treatment; each time it should become less painful. By the second treatment, the congestion causing such areas to be oversensitive should have begun to disperse.

BELOW *Most people find the treatment extremely relaxing. Particularly sensitive areas should become less painful with subsequent treatments.*

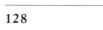

TREATMENT EFFECTS

By the end of the treatment, you may feel a warm glow over the whole body, or you may feel quite light and often completely free of pain. On a psychological level, after treatment you may feel euphoric, or be in a deeply relaxed state. The effects may not last until the next treatment, but chronic symptoms often return with less intensity, and over successive treatments the period of freedom from discomfort lengthens and the problem should gradually be alleviated.

It is not possible to ascertain the number of treatment sessions needed, as each client and disorder are individual. Most people find that they begin to improve noticeably after three to six treatments, though many find some relief after only one visit. Clients may also be shown how to apply self-help treatment in between sessions, as this provides ongoing therapeutic stimulation. After the initial period, a practitioner will probably extend your treatment intervals from weekly to alternate weeks, then to monthly or six-weekly; some people need only two treatments per year.

ELLEN MASTERS
REFLEXOLOGIST

Client's name: *Kevin Shaw*

Your next appointment with the reflexologist will be on

Date: *26th August*

LEFT *After an initial period, your treatment interval will probably extend from weekly to monthly intervals.*

REACTIONS TO TREATMENT

After the treatment session, it is quite normal to get a response. For instance, there may be an increase in bowel action and urination. Or you may have a heavy head or aching limbs; this is a result of toxins that have been released into your system. They can be eliminated by increasing your water intake. Some people find that they experience a temporary outbreak of acne or a slight skin irritation.

Emotional reactions can take many forms: agitation, anger, anxiety, distress, or laughter, and form an important release. Although symptoms of any disorder may be slightly exacerbated in the first 24 hours, after this, if any symptom seems worse, contact your medical practitioner. The term "healing crisis" is often used in many books, but there is no crisis with reflexology. The above reactions are a normal outcome of treatment and often show that a positive effect has been achieved. Reflexology treatment is a totally noninvasive natural therapy aimed at a restoration of health.

LEFT *The hands may also be worked on during a treatment session.*

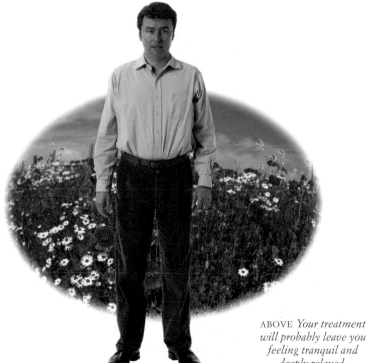

ABOVE *Your treatment will probably leave you feeling tranquil and deeply relaxed.*

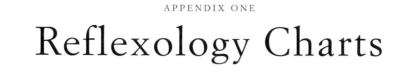

APPENDIX ONE
Reflexology Charts

REFLEX AREAS OF THE FOOT – SOLES OF THE FEET

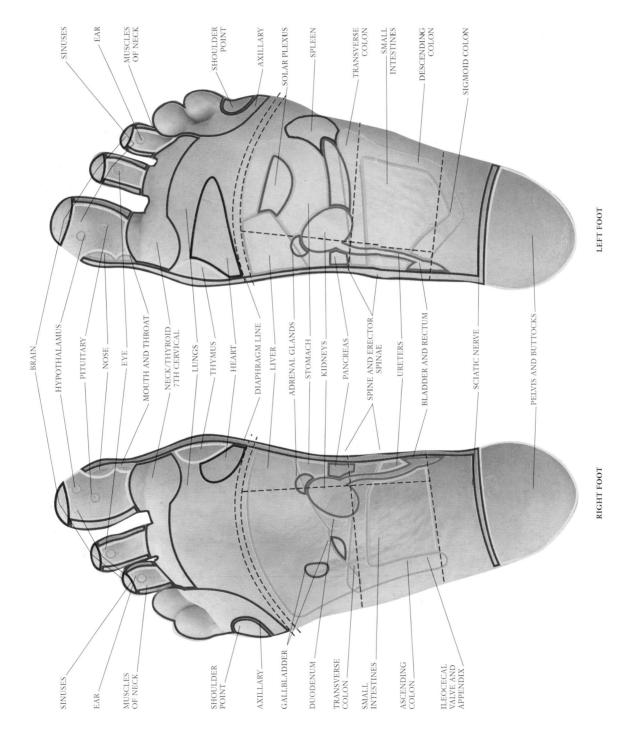

REFLEX AREAS OF THE FOOT – DORSAL VIEW OF THE FEET

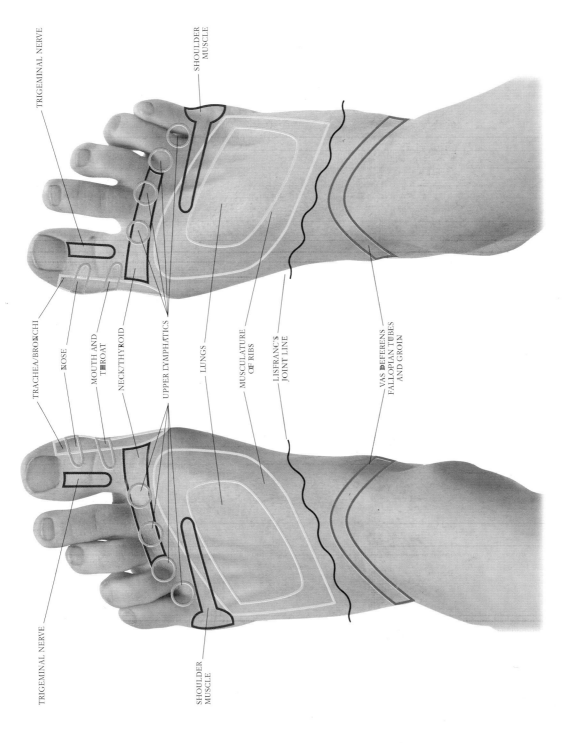

RIGHT FOOT

LEFT FOOT

TRIGEMINAL NERVE

SHOULDER MUSCLE

TRACHEA/BRONCHI

NOSE

MOUTH AND THROAT

NECK/THYROID

UPPER LYMPHATICS

LUNGS

MUSCULATURE OF RIBS

LISFRANC'S JOINT LINE

VAS DEFERENS FALLOPIAN TUBES AND GROIN

TRIGEMINAL NERVE

SHOULDER MUSCLE

REFLEX AREAS OF THE FOOT – OUTER AND INNER ASPECTS OF FOOT

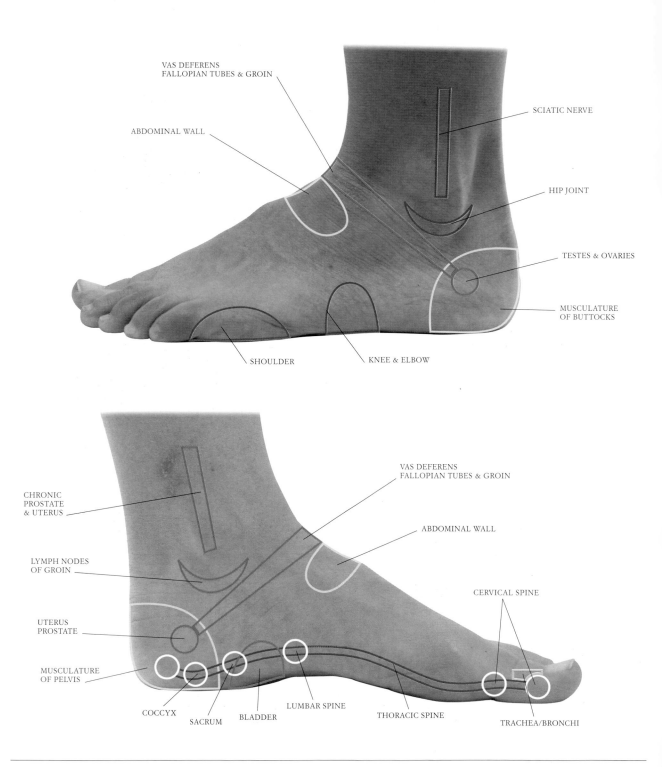

VAS DEFERENS
FALLOPIAN TUBES & GROIN

ABDOMINAL WALL

SCIATIC NERVE

HIP JOINT

TESTES & OVARIES

MUSCULATURE
OF BUTTOCKS

SHOULDER

KNEE & ELBOW

CHRONIC
PROSTATE
& UTERUS

VAS DEFERENS
FALLOPIAN TUBES & GROIN

ABDOMINAL WALL

LYMPH NODES
OF GROIN

CERVICAL SPINE

UTERUS
PROSTATE

MUSCULATURE
OF PELVIS

COCCYX

SACRUM

BLADDER

LUMBAR SPINE

THORACIC SPINE

TRACHEA/BRONCHI

REFLEX AREAS OF THE THE PALMAR SURFACE OF THE HANDS

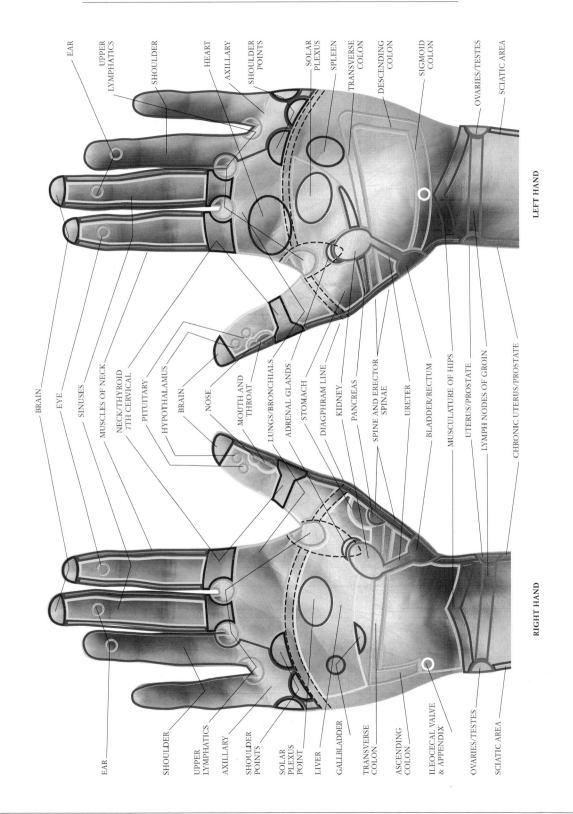

LEFT HAND

RIGHT HAND

EAR
UPPER LYMPHATICS
SHOULDER
HEART
AXILLARY
SHOULDER POINTS
SOLAR PLEXUS
SPLEEN
TRANSVERSE COLON
DESCENDING COLON
SIGMOID COLON
OVARIES/TESTES
SCIATIC AREA

BRAIN
EYE
SINUSES
MUSCLES OF NECK
NECK/THYROID 7TH CERVICAL
PITUITARY
HYPOTHALAMUS
BRAIN
NOSE
MOUTH AND THROAT
LUNGS/BRONCHIALS
ADRENAL GLANDS
STOMACH
DIAGPHRAM LINE
KIDNEY
PANCREAS
SPINE AND ERECTOR SPINAE
URETER
BLADDER/RECTUM
MUSCULATURE OF HIPS
UTERUS/PROSTATE
LYMPH NODES OF GROIN
CHRONIC UTERUS/PROSTATE

EAR
SHOULDER
UPPER LYMPHATICS
AXILLARY
SHOULDER POINTS
SOLAR PLEXUS POINT
LIVER
GALLBLADDER
TRANSVERSE COLON
ASCENDING COLON
ILEOCECAL VALVE & APPENDIX
OVARIES/TESTES
SCIATIC AREA

REFLEX AREAS OF THE DORSAL SURFACE OF THE HANDS

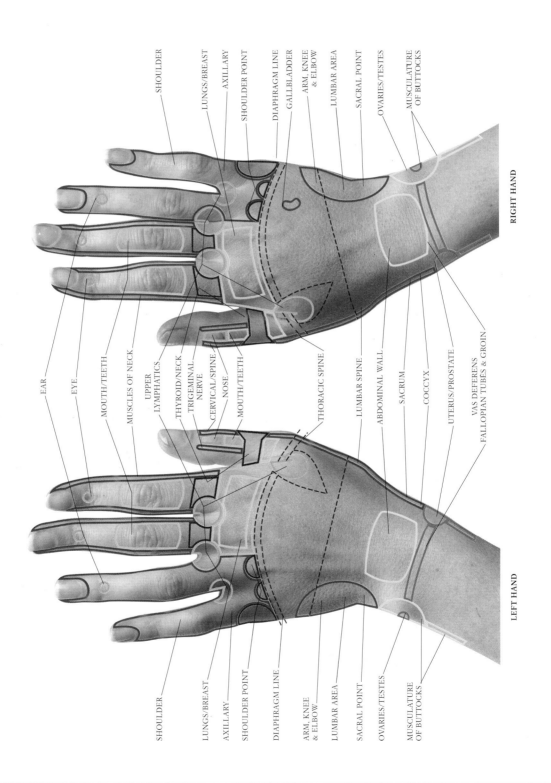

RIGHT HAND

LEFT HAND

SHOULDER
LUNGS/BREAST
AXILLARY
SHOULDER POINT
DIAPHRAGM LINE
GALLBLADDER
ARM, KNEE & ELBOW
LUMBAR AREA
SACRAL POINT
OVARIES/TESTES
MUSCULATURE OF BUTTOCKS

EAR
EYE
MOUTH/TEETH
MUSCLES OF NECK
UPPER LYMPHATICS
THYROID/NECK
TRIGEMINAL NERVE
CERVICAL/SPINE
NOSE
MOUTH/TEETH
THORACIC SPINE
LUMBAR SPINE
ABDOMINAL WALL
SACRUM
COCCYX
UTERUS/PROSTATE
VAS DEFERENS
FALLOPIAN TUBES & GROIN

SHOULDER
LUNGS/BREAST
AXILLARY
SHOULDER POINT
DIAPHRAGM LINE
ARM, KNEE & ELBOW
LUMBAR AREA
SACRAL POINT
OVARIES/TESTES
MUSCULATURE OF BUTTOCKS

REFLEX AREAS OF THE EAR

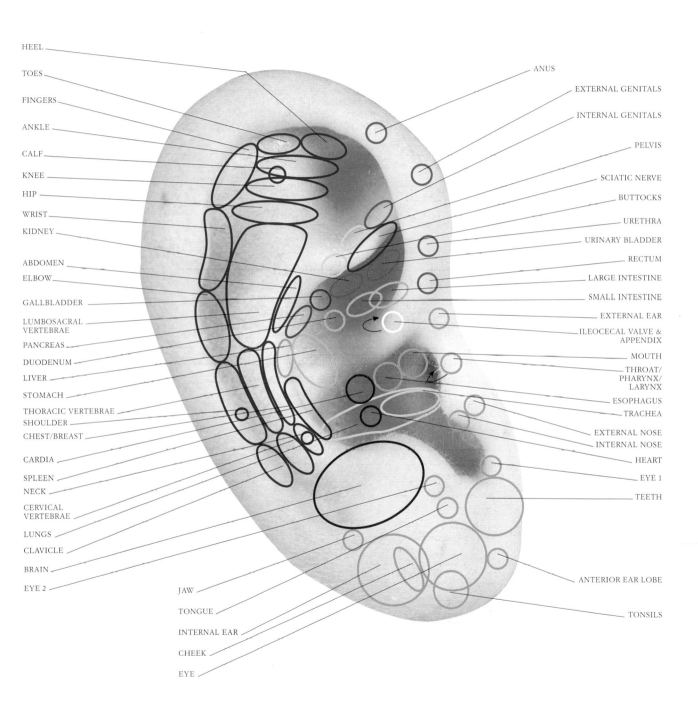

HEEL

TOES

FINGERS

ANKLE

CALF

KNEE

HIP

WRIST

KIDNEY

ABDOMEN

ELBOW

GALLBLADDER

LUMBOSACRAL
VERTEBRAE

PANCREAS

DUODENUM

LIVER

STOMACH

THORACIC VERTEBRAE

SHOULDER

CHEST/BREAST

CARDIA

SPLEEN

NECK

CERVICAL
VERTEBRAE

LUNGS

CLAVICLE

BRAIN

EYE 2

JAW

TONGUE

INTERNAL EAR

CHEEK

EYE

ANUS

EXTERNAL GENITALS

INTERNAL GENITALS

PELVIS

SCIATIC NERVE

BUTTOCKS

URETHRA

URINARY BLADDER

RECTUM

LARGE INTESTINE

SMALL INTESTINE

EXTERNAL EAR

ILEOCECAL VALVE &
APPENDIX

MOUTH

THROAT/
PHARYNX/
LARYNX

ESOPHAGUS

TRACHEA

EXTERNAL NOSE

INTERNAL NOSE

HEART

EYE 1

TEETH

ANTERIOR EAR LOBE

TONSILS

APPENDIX TWO

The Chinese Meridians

YIN MERIDIANS OF THE LEG

KEY

SP-1 great toe, medial edge of the nail bed

SP-2 in the middle of the lower bone on the great toe

SP-3 at the distal end of the first metatarsals – the inner arch at the front of the foot

SP-4 at the proximal end of the first (metatarsal) foot bone

SP-5 in the depression in front of the inner ankle

SP-6 4 finger-widths above the inside ankle bone, just behind the tibia (shin bone)

SP-9 in the depression below the head of the tibia

LIV-2 at the base of the web between the big and second toe

LIV-3 in the furrow between the big and second toes

KI-1 in the middle of the crease just behind the ball of the foot

KI-2 on the inner foot, just below the navicular bone
(See Structure of Foot and Hand, p. 45.)

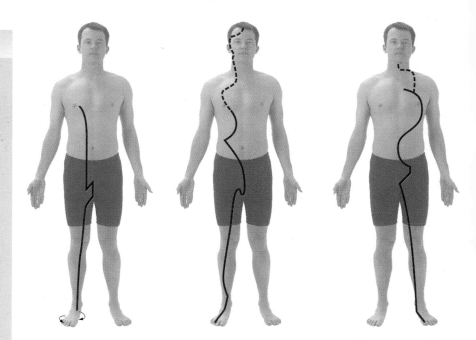

KIDNEY MERIDIAN   LIVER MERIDIAN   SPLEEN/PANCREAS MERIDIAN

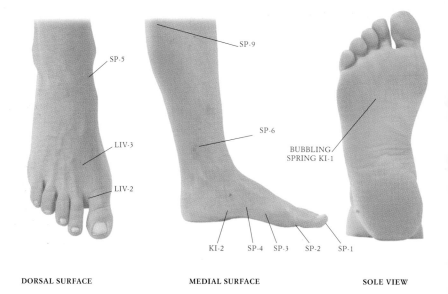

DORSAL SURFACE   MEDIAL SURFACE   SOLE VIEW

YANG MERIDIANS OF THE LEG

KEY

ST-35 beside the kneecap

ST-36 4 finger-widths below the kneecap, outside the tibia bone

ST-39 in the middle of the lower leg

ST-40 6 finger-widths below ST-36.

ST-44 on top of the foot in the web between the second and third toes

ST-45 at the base of the second toe nail bed

BL-60 around lateral ankle bone

BL-63 on the outer edge of the foot just below the ankle

BL-66 on first bone of the little toe

GB-14 one finger-width above the midline of each eyebrow

GB-37 6 finger-widths above the outside ankle bone on the side of the lower leg, in front of the fibula bone

GB-41 in the furrow between the fourth and fifth toe, as far up as you can go in the channel between the bones

GB-42 on the top of the foot in the furrow between the fourth and fifth toes

GB-44 on the nail bed of the fourth toe, outside edge

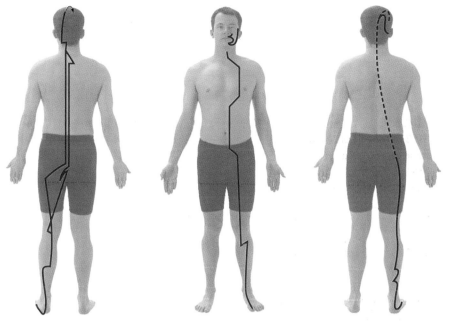

BLADDER MERIDIAN

STOMACH MERIDIAN

GALLBLADDER MERIDIAN

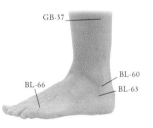

GB-37

BL-66

BL-60

BL-63

LATERAL SURFACE

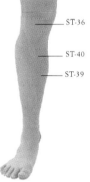

ST-35

ST-36

ST-40

ST-39

FRONT VIEW

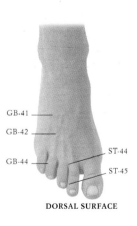

GB-41

GB-42

GB-44

ST-44

ST-45

DORSAL SURFACE

CAUTION

Do not use BL-60 in pregnancy, since this point is used for placental retention. Therefore one can see why it should not be worked in pregnancy.

YIN MERIDIANS OF THE ARM

KEY

LU-8 just above the wrist crease, on the thumb side

LU-9 on the wrist crease, thumb side

LU-10 2 thumb-widths below the wrist crease on the thumb pad

LU-11 on the thumb, on the outside corner of the nail bed

HE-4 2 finger-widths above the wrist crease, little-finger side of the inner forearm

HE-5 1 thumb-width above the wrist crease

HE-6 half a thumbs-width above the wrist crease

HE-7 (Shenmen) on the wrist crease

HE-8 in line with the base of the thumb web below the fourth or little fingers

HE-9 on the inside tip of the little finger

PE-4 1 hands-width above the wrist, on the inner forearm

PE-5 4 finger-widths up from the wrist crease

PE-6 2 thumb-widths up from the wrist crease

PE-7 on wrist crease

PE-8 palm, below the second finger or big finger

PE-9 at the tip of the second finger or big finger

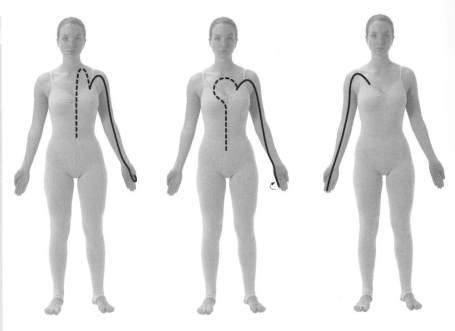

LUNG MERIDIAN   HEART MERIDIAN   PERICARDIUM MERIDIAN

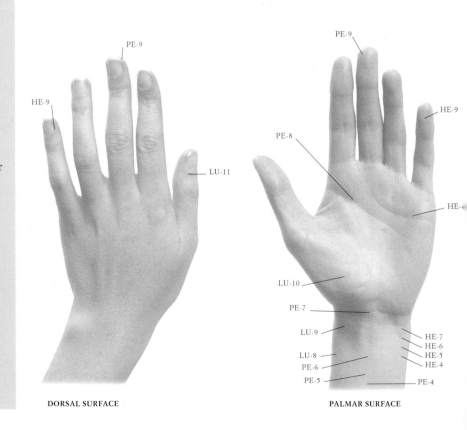

DORSAL SURFACE

PALMAR SURFACE

YANG MERIDIANS OF THE ARM

KEY

LI-1 at the nail bed of the index finger, thumb side

LI-2 at the base of the proximal phalange

LI-3 at the base of the first finger, thumb side

LI-4 in the web of the thumb and index finger

LI-20 in the nose crease as you smile, as near to the nose as possible

TB-1 at the base of the third finger nail bed

TB-2 in the web between the third and fourth fingers

TB-3 on the back of the hand, between the fourth and fifth knuckles

TB-4 in the depression of the wrist

TB-5 in the middle of the back of the forearm, 2 thumb-widths above the wrist crease

TB-6 4 thumb-widths up from the wrist crease

TB-23 on the outside edge side of each eyebrow

SI-1 on the outside edge of the nail bed on the little finger

SI-2 at the base of the little finger, outer edge

SI-3 on the knuckle beneath the little finger, outer edge

SI-4 at the base of the fifth hand bone

SI-5 in the hollow of the wrist joint

SI-19 in the depression formed next to the ear when you open your mouth

CAUTION

The point LI-4 must not be used during pregnancy, although it may be used during labor.

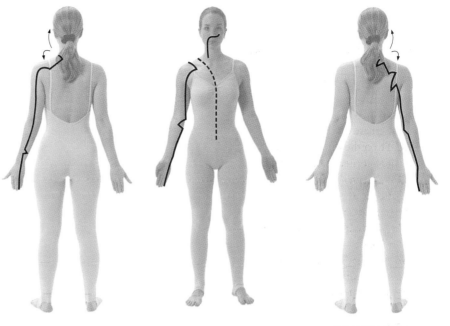

TRIPLE BURNER MERIDIAN

LARGE INTESTINE MERIDIAN

SMALL INTESTINE MERIDIAN

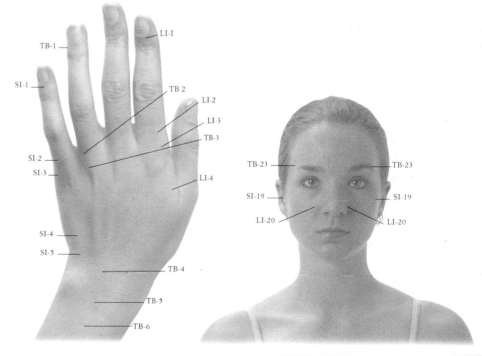

DORSAL SURFACE

FACIAL PRESSURE POINTS

THE CONCEPTION AND GOVERNOR VESSELS

KEY

ST-1 on the bone just below the eye, in line with pupil

ST-2 immediately below ST-1

BL-1 in the depression just above the inner corner of each eye

BL-2 on inner edge of each eyebrow

BL-10 on hairline of the neck, two finger-widths either side of, spine

GB-1 on the outer corner of the eye

GB-20 (Fengchi) either side of the nape of the neck, above the hair line

GB-21 in the depression on the shoulders in line with ears

GV-26 in the midline directly under the nose

GV-20 (Baihui) on the highest point of the head

GV-19 2 finger-widths below

GV-16 in the center of the nape of the neck, just above the hair line

CV-24 on the middle of the lower lip

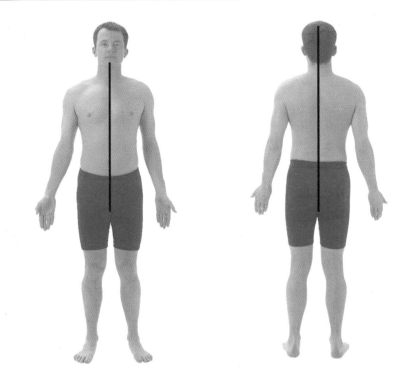

CONCEPTION VESSEL   GOVERNOR VESSEL

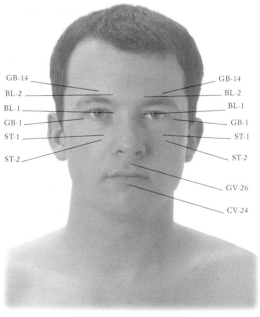

FACIAL PRESSURE POINTS

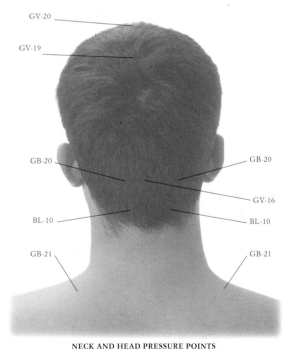

NECK AND HEAD PRESSURE POINTS

Bibliography and Further Reading

ARNOT, Michelle, *Foot Notes,* Sphere Books, London, 1982

BAYLY, Doreen, *Reflexology Today,* Thorsons, New York, 1986

BRESSLER, Harry Bond, *Zone Therapy,* Health Research, Mokelumne Hill, California, 1971

CRANE, Beryl, *Reflexology: The Definitive Practitioner's Manual,* Element Books, 1997

DOUGANS, Inge, *Complete Illustrated Guide to Reflexology,* Element Books, 1996

FITZGERALD, William H. and Bowers, Edwin F., *Zone Therapy,* Health Research, Mokelumne Hill, California, 1917

HALL, Nicola M., *Reflexology – A Way to Better Health,* Pan Books, London, 1988

ISSEL, Christine, *Reflexology: Art, Science and History,* New Frontier Publishing, Sacramento, 1990

Useful Addresses

EUROPE

Denmark
FORENEDE DANSKE ZONETERAPEUTER
FDZ Secretariat,
Chr. Winthersvej 13,
DK 6000 Kolding ,
Denmark
Tel 45 7550 1250
Fax 45 7550 7447

Finland
FINNISH ASSOCIATION OF NATURAL THERAPIES
Pilspan,
Kylantle,
01730 Vantaa,
Finland
Tel 358 9276 7424

Germany
DEUTSCHER REFLEXOLOGEN VERBAND
Lloyd G. Wells Str. 15,
14163 Berlin,
Germany
Tel 49 30 813 10 22
Fax 49 30 813 10 27

Italy
FEDERATZIONE ITALIANA DI REFLESSOLOGIA DEL PIEDE
Via Rinaldini Nio Bis,
Vestone,
Bresica 25078

Netherlands
BOND VAN EUROPESE REFLEXOLOGEN (Society of European Reflexologists)
Netherlands Section
PO Box 9009,
1006 AA Amsterdam,
Netherlands
Fax 31 34 20 22178/
31 20 61 76918

UK
ASSOCIATION OF REFLEXOLOGISTS
23 Old Gloucester Street,
London WC1N 3XX
Tel 0990 673320

THE CRANE SCHOOL OF REFLEXOLOGY
135 Collins Meadow,
Harrow,
Essex CH19 4ES
Tel 01279 421682
Fax 01279 441304

REFLEXOLOGIST'S SOCIETY
249 Fosse Road South
Leicester
LE3 9PG

COUNTRIES OUTSIDE EUROPE

Australia
REFLEXOLOGY ASSOCIATION OF AUSTRALIA
PO Box 366
Cammeray
New South Wales 2062,
Australia

Canada
REFLEXOLOGY ASSOCIATION OF CANADA (RAC)
Box 110
541 Tumberry Street
Brussels,
Ontario N0G 1HO,
Canada
Tel 1 510 887 9991
Fax 1 510 887 9792

China
CHINA REFLEXOLOGY ASSOCIATION
PO Box 2002,
Beijing 100026,
China
Tel 86 10 5068310
Fax 86 10 5068309

Japan
REFLEXOLOGY ASSOCIATION OF JAPAN
Akasaka TS Building, 5-1-36
Akasaka
Minato-ky
Tokyo 107

Russia
I M SECHENOV MOSCOW MEDICAL ACADEMY
Dept of Complementary Medicine,
B. Pirogovskaja 2/6,
Moscow 119881,
Russia
Tel 7 095 246 96676
Fax 7 095 248 0214

South Africa
THE SOUTH AFRICAN REFLEXOLOGY SOCIETY
PO Box 201858,
Durban North 4016,
South Africa

United States
REFLEXOLOGY ASSOCIATION OF CALIFORNIA
PO Box 641156,
Los Angeles,
California 90064

REFLEXOLOGY ASSOCIATION OF AMERICA
4012 S. Rainbow Boulevard,
Box K585,
Las Vegas,
Nevada 89103-2509

Index